NUMERACY
AND CLINICAL CALCULATIONS
FOR NURSES
SECOND EDITION

Key titles for new nurses

Pocket Guides series

Each of these unique books provides a wealth of practical detail, tips and advice to help you get to grips with, and make the most of, your placements.

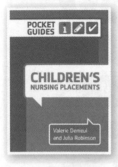 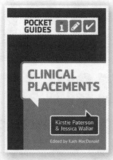 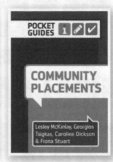 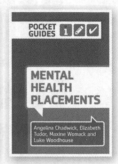

Essentials series

Practical introductory textbooks featuring clear explanations, scenarios, activities and case studies. They will help you learn the subject quickly and easily.

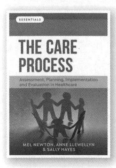 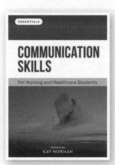 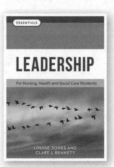 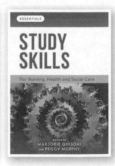

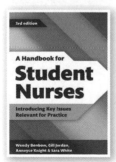

A Handbook for Student Nurses provides an introduction to the essential background knowledge that you need as a foundation for your pre-registration training, including:

- Practice supervision and assessment
- Communication
- Legal and professional issues
- Values, ethics and cultural awareness
- Reflection and personal development
- Quality care and evidence-based practice
- Study skills
- Public health and promoting health and wellbeing

NUMERACY AND CLINICAL CALCULATIONS FOR NURSES

SECOND EDITION

Neil Davison

Teaching Fellow, Bangor University

Lantern

ISBN: 9781908625793

Second edition published 2020

First edition published 2015 by Lantern Publishing Limited (ISBN 9781908625243); reprinted 2015, 2016, 2017, 2018

Lantern Publishing Limited, The Old Hayloft, Vantage Business Park, Bloxham Rd, Banbury, OX16 9UX, UK

www.lanternpublishing.com

www.cla.co.uk

British Library Cataloguing in Publication Data

A catalogue record for this book is available from the British Library

The authors and publisher have made every attempt to ensure the content of this book is up to date and accurate. However, healthcare knowledge and information is changing all the time so the reader is advised to double-check any information in this text on drug usage, treatment procedures, the use of equipment, etc. to confirm that it complies with the latest safety recommendations, standards of practice and legislation, as well as local Trust policies and procedures. Students are advised to check with their tutor and/or practice supervisor before carrying out any of the procedures in this textbook.

Typeset by Medlar Publishing Solutions Pvt Ltd, India

Cover design by Andrew Magee Design Ltd

Printed in the UK

Last digit is the print number: 10 9 8 7 6 5 4 3

CONTENTS

ABOUT THE AUTHOR

Neil Davison worked in trauma and orthopaedics after the completion of his state registration and orthopaedic nursing qualifications in the 1970s and early 1980s. He lectured at Bangor University for two decades and has extensive experience of teaching drug calculations and numeracy to both pre- and post-registration students. He was made a Teaching Fellow at the university in 1999 and retired in 2012. Since then Neil has continued to teach on healthcare courses in the further education sector and in the hospitals of North Wales.

PREFACE TO THE SECOND EDITION

Drug and clinical calculations are a significant part of modern nursing practice but performing them can cause unnecessary anxiety in many nurses.

This drug calculation book is written for student nurses at the start of their career and registered nurses who need a refresher. It is influenced by many years of teaching numeracy and drug calculation skills to undergraduate nurses in the classroom and practice setting, preparing them for online and traditional examinations and ultimately registration with the NMC.

The book aims to increase the reader's skills and confidence in calculating drug doses, whether in preparation for clinical practice, drug calculation exams or as part of professional updating. This is achieved by an initial self-assessment of numeracy skills, followed by practical examples that explore the key principles, techniques and formulae needed to accurately calculate drug dosages. This second edition provides more opportunities to assess your progress throughout the book and additional comprehensive summary tests in the final chapter.

Neil Davison

ACKNOWLEDGEMENTS

The publishers would like to thank the following lecturers and a selection of their students for reviewing the Back to Basics chapter of this book and providing useful comments that have informed the final version:

Maureen Crowley, University of the West of Scotland
David Maynard, Birmingham City University
Caroline Ridley, Manchester Metropolitan University
Maggie Roberts, University of Nottingham

Thanks also to Judy Waterlow for permission to reproduce the Waterlow chart (www.judy-waterlow.co.uk).

The 'Malnutrition Universal Screening Tool' ('MUST') is reproduced with the kind permission of BAPEN (British Association for Parenteral and Enteral Nutrition). For further information on 'MUST' see www.bapen.org.uk.

The National Early Warning Score (NEWS) is reproduced with permission from the Royal College of Physicians. *National Early Warning Score (NEWS) 2: Standardising the assessment of acute-illness severity in the NHS*. Updated report of a working party. London: RCP, 2017.

HOW TO USE THIS BOOK

There are various ways to use this book:

If you are a student nurse or have returned to nursing after a career break and want a comprehensive understanding of drug and clinical calculations used in nursing, then read the book cover to cover.

If you are confident in your basic numeracy skills but want to learn how to apply these to the clinical setting, concentrate on *Chapters 3 to 6*. These will equip you with information about the SI system used in healthcare, how to calculate drug doses and the use of numbers and calculations in other areas of clinical practice like nutrition and fluid balance. *Chapter 6* contains several tests so you can check your knowledge and understanding.

If you are an experienced nurse and have changed career directions and are unsure whether your current knowledge of drug and clinical calculations is up to scratch, then focus your study on *Chapters 3, 4* and *6*. This will allow you to revise the SI system and practise calculating drug doses and other clinical calculations.

If you are confident in your basic numeracy skills but want to gain more practice of drug calculations then concentrate your efforts on *Chapters 3, 4* and *6*. These focus mainly on drugs, the units of measurement and calculating correct doses.

If you are revising for a drug calculation exam, focus on *Chapters 3, 4* and *6*. These chapters explain the SI system and the fundamentals of calculating drug doses as well as providing many clinically related practice calculations.

01

NUMERACY AND CALCULATION SKILLS IN THE CLINICAL ENVIRONMENT

THIS CHAPTER:

- concentrates on why you need calculation and numeracy skills

- considers common sources of drug and calculation errors

- identifies the various opportunities available to help you learn (or re-learn) the necessary calculation skills

- has a self-assessment test at the end, so that you can identify your strengths and diagnose your weaknesses.

1.1 Why you need to know about numbers and calculations

As a nurse, you will be required to deal with numbers and perform basic calculations every day, for example:

- ensuring accurate administration of drugs

- completing a fluid balance chart

- calculating a BMI.

It is therefore absolutely crucial, for you and for your patients, that you become confident in handling numbers and familiar with the calculations you will come across in your practice. By doing this, you will help to ensure that your patients get the best and safest care possible from the healthcare services and from you. Nursing is, in part, about 'doing things right and doing the right things' and drug and clinical calculations are an integral part of everyday nursing. 'Doing things right' is about ensuring the accuracy of your calculations, and 'doing the right things' is then applying your numeracy and calculation skills to the variety of situations that depend on it.

The Nursing and Midwifery Council (NMC) considers numeracy skills to be a part of being an accountable professional. The *Standards of Proficiency for Registered Nurses* indicate that the areas of practice underpinned by numeracy skills go beyond performing drug calculations and administering medicines to include several areas of patient assessment and nutritional and fluid support.

To register with the NMC, students will need to pass a health numeracy assessment related to nursing proficiencies and calculation of medicines, with a score of 100%. If you are already a registered nurse and are refreshing and updating your numeracy skills, this gives you a clear indication of the standards expected of new registrants and the level of skill that you need to achieve.

The UK population is ageing and many of the patients you will deal with will be older and have complex needs; this frequently means that patients need more drugs, intravenous fluids and care assessments, all of which require numeracy and calculation skills. It is estimated that a typical registered nurse will spend up to a third of each working day on some aspect of the medication administration process (Keers *et al.*, 2013), even before taking account of other calculations such as fluid balance charts or weighing patients. In view of the changing needs of patients, the amount of time that nurses spend performing calculations is only likely to increase year by year.

Apart from the day-to-day performance in your health care role, you will need to be confident and familiar with calculations and numbers as many employers now use a numeracy test as part of the selection and recruitment process. In addition, mandatory annual updating and testing of numeracy skills is becoming a more common feature of nurses' personal and professional development.

1.2 Common calculation errors

Whenever there is a calculation to be made, there is a possibility of an error. Knowing the situations where mistakes are more likely to be made and the type of calculation errors means that you are more alert to these possibilities, and hopefully less likely to fall into the trap.

Mistakes made with drug and clinical calculations usually involve:

- getting the maths wrong
- getting the dosage unit wrong
- communication errors.

Getting the maths wrong

Chapter 2 deals with the mechanics of performing calculations and the use of decimal points as well as providing plenty of questions with which to test yourself.

- A basic calculation mistake caused the death of a patient in Scotland in 2005. The nurse failed to get her dosage calculation checked by a colleague and she gave 40 units of insulin to a patient instead of the prescribed 4 units.

- A mathematical miscalculation by two nurses working in a Leicestershire hospital caused the death of a baby in 2002. The nurses both made the same error with a decimal point, resulting in the baby receiving ten times more of a drug than was intended.

Getting the dosage unit wrong

Chapter 3 focuses on the SI system used throughout the UK. It is used to ensure that standardised sets of units are used for weights and volumes of medicines and fluids in healthcare.

- In two separate Scottish nursing homes 'International Unit' had been shortened to 'IU'. A prescription for 6 units of insulin became 6IU, resulting in the patients receiving 61 units.

Communication errors

Communication is a vital part of healthcare and the quality and accuracy of writing is a source of calculation mistakes.

- In 2005, a baby died in a Liverpool hospital after being given 15 000 units of the anticoagulant heparin instead of the prescribed 1500 units. The hand-written prescription read 1500U and the nurse mistook the 'U', wrongly used as an abbreviation for units, for a zero.

ERROR ALERT

Carefully reading a prescription is essential:
In 2017, in a hospital in the north of England, a patient had been prescribed **oxybutynin** 5 mg, which is a medication used to regulate urinary frequency. A nurse mistakenly administered **oxycontin** 5 mg to the patient. Oxycontin, an opioid painkiller, is a controlled drug.

ERROR ALERT

Sometimes, what appears to be a drug calculation error isn't.

- At a West Midlands hospital in 2011, a nurse gave a patient ten times the amount of prescribed potassium chloride, an electrolyte that influences the heart rate and contraction. Predictably the patient suffered a fatal cardiac arrest.
- The nurse had calculated the correct dose but did not get another nurse to witness the administration of the drug.
- If another nurse had observed the administration (as demanded by the checking procedure), it would have become apparent that the infusion pump was set up wrongly, allowing it to give ten times the prescribed dose.
- This catastrophic series of events, resulting in a patient death, was because of an administration error, not a calculation mistake.
- Numeracy skills are essential in nursing, but following standardised procedures and being proficient in the use of medical devices that control drug administration are of equal importance.

1.3 Developing your calculation and numeracy skills

Having scared you by describing the worst possible outcomes of calculation errors, I will now ask you not to get overly anxious about making a mistake! Concerns about nurses' calculation skills have featured in the literature since 1939, and span the globe, so this isn't a recent problem or one that only occurs in the UK. But drug and calculation errors are currently widely reported, probably because mistakes in the prescribing and administration of drugs account for 25% of litigation claims in the UK, and government pledges to reduce this by 40% have failed. More importantly, these kinds of mistakes are of serious concern to healthcare consumers and in the aftermath of the Francis report (2013) into the failings at the Mid-Staffordshire NHS Foundation Trust, they could be seen as a quality indicator. Remember though that drug calculation errors are rare.

Fortunately, there are many methods and techniques to ensure that your calculation and numeracy skills are robust, safe and fit for modern clinical practice. Good starting points include:

- reading this book

- taking the self-tests

- practising calculations.

The theory part of calculations is covered within undergraduate courses leading to registration and revised on nurse prescribing and similar courses. Like any skill, it is important to practise and taking self-tests is a large part of this. Numeracy skills are an essential clinical skill, so expect to practise these alongside your other clinical skills.

Before starting on a clinical placement:

- Spend a few minutes thinking about the potential opportunities that lie ahead.

- Remember that patient assessment and admission, taking and recording physiological observation like temperature, pulse and blood pressure and recording a fluid intake and output chart all demand calculation skills apart from administering medicines.

If you are unsure of the learning opportunities available on your next clinical placement and how these might allow you to practise calculations:

- Talk to the Link tutor from your university.

- Talk to other students who may have spent time on the placement.

- Visit the placement and meet with your mentor before starting.

There may be a booklet for students outlining typical learning opportunities. Aim to make the most of every minute of your clinical experience. Working alongside an experienced nurse and getting involved in drug rounds will help you develop the required calculation skills, as well as help you to become familiar with common drug doses and to recognise when something isn't right.

Self-assessment test 1.1

To help you identify a baseline where you are starting from, try the following self-assessment test, using pencil and paper where necessary but not a calculator. The NMC standards dictate that registered nurses must be able to perform calculations without the use of a calculator. If you are unable to answer some of the questions don't worry, as the whole purpose of this book is to increase your understanding of drug and clinical calculations.

Once you have completed the test, check your answers with the answer section at the end of the book. The feedback and suggested actions below will give you advice about which chapters and sections you need to focus on to develop your numeracy and calculation skills.

Self-assessment test 1.1 (*continued*)

1 25 + 34 =

2 Write 1005 in words.

3 Which of the following numbers is the larger, 2858 or 28580?

4 56 − 24 =

5 What does the zero in 860 mean?

6 5 × 9 =

7 How many more is 104 than 97?

8 74 + 87 =

9 Write out 960012 in words.

10 6 × 8 =

11 105 − 76 =

12 What does the 5 in 2450198 mean?

13 9 × 12 =

14 How many more is 1204 than 89?

15 If you scored 80 out of a possible 125 in a test, what percentage did you achieve?

16 14 × 18 =

17 What does the zero in 19061 mean?

18 115 / 8 =

19 How many micrograms are there in 0.65 milligrams?

20 Write 80% as a fraction.

21 1.61 × 2.38 =

22 How many grams are there in 0.823 kilograms?

23 102 − 78 =

24 Write 0.75 as a percentage.

25 5.912 × 8.647 =

26 1.643 × 0.724 =

27 How many milligrams are there in 1.2 grams?

28 Which of these fractions is the larger, ⅔ or ¾?

29 Write 55% as a decimal.

30 How many millilitres are there in 0.006 litres?

Feedback and suggested actions

If you made a mistake or had any difficulty with questions 1 or 8, you'll find more guidance about this in *Chapter 2* in the 'Addition' section.

If questions 4, 11 or 23 gave you problems, the 'Subtraction' section in *Chapter 2* should help you.

If questions 6, 10, 13 or 16 caused you any difficulties, the section in *Chapter 2* on 'Multiplication' should provide you with the techniques and practice questions to overcome these.

If question 18 caused problems, go to the 'Division' section of *Chapter 2*.

If you had problems with questions 2, 5, 9, 12 or 17, go to 'The decimal system' section in *Chapter 2*.

If questions 3, 7 or 14 tripped you up, start your reading at the beginning of *Chapter 2* where you'll find more information.

Questions 15, 20, 24, 28 and 29 related to fractions and percentages. If any of these questions gave you problems, the sections on 'Fractions' and 'Percentages' in *Chapter 2* should give you the information to put this right.

If questions 19, 22, 27 or 30 caused concerns, you'll find more information in *Chapter 3*, 'The SI System'.

Questions 21, 25 and 26 involved multiplying decimals. If these got you scratching your head then reading the 'Multiplying decimals' section in *Chapter 2* should help.

If you were able to answer most of the self-assessment test questions without too much trouble, start by reading *Chapter 3*. This explains the SI system of measurement in more detail. Then move on to *Chapter 4* that considers how to calculate drug doses and then progress to *Chapter 5* on other clinical calculations. *Chapter 6* will give you the opportunity to put your knowledge to the test.

KEY POINTS TO TAKE AWAY FROM THIS CHAPTER

- Nurses need accurate calculation skills and a solid knowledge of numeracy for the safe administration of drugs and many other parts of their daily work.
- Calculation errors are rare and can be prevented with practice and care.
- There are many opportunities to develop your calculation skills during the theory and practice parts of your course.

02

BACK TO BASICS

THIS CHAPTER:

- gives an overview of the decimal system
- revises the four basic methods of calculating
- considers ways of expressing and calculating numbers less than one
- describes how very large numbers can be expressed.

2.1 Introduction

The modern healthcare environment demands a good understanding of decimals and the ability to use them. This includes whole numbers like 18, 140 and 567 as well as parts of whole numbers. Some medications are prescribed in whole numbers, for example paracetamol 500 mg, and some are prescribed in amounts that include less than one unit, for example bendroflumethiazide 2.5 mg.

2.2 The decimal system

A number is made up from individual digits and communicates a great deal of information. If 475 is used as an example, this isn't simply a '4', a '7' and a '5'. The place of the digit within the number gives a value such as hundreds, tens and ones. Reading from left to right 475 has a value of 4 'hundreds', 7 'tens' and 5 'ones'. This is because we use a 'base 10' decimal system. This means that the value of each place in a number is 10 times greater than the number to the right of it. The place value of '7' is tens and of '5' is ones. Similarly, the value of each place is ten times smaller than the place to its left. *Figure 2.1* presents this visually.

MILLIONS	HUNDRED THOUSANDS	TEN THOUSANDS	THOUSANDS	HUNDREDS	TENS	ONES/UNITS	DECIMAL POINT	TENTHS	HUNDREDTHS	THOUSANDTHS
1 000 000	100 000	10 000	1000	100	10	1	.	0.1	0.01	0.001
WHOLE NUMBERS TO THE LEFT OF THE DECIMAL POINT							.	DECIMAL FRACTIONS TO THE RIGHT OF THE DECIMAL POINT		

Figure 2.1. *Whole numbers and decimal fractions.*

Using the example of digoxin (a drug used to control an irregular heart rate), a common dosage is 125 micrograms. The place values in the number tell us the exact amount to give: 1 'hundred', 2 'tens' and 5 'ones' or 'one hundred and twenty-five' micrograms. *Figure 2.2* illustrates this.

MILLIONS	HUNDRED THOUSANDS	TEN THOUSANDS	THOUSANDS	HUNDREDS	TENS	ONES/UNITS	DECIMAL POINT	TENTHS	HUNDREDTHS	THOUSANDTHS
				1	2	5				

Figure 2.2. *Digoxin 125 micrograms.*

The decimal point is used to signpost the end of the whole number and the beginning of amounts that are less than one. Returning to the digoxin example, this can also be prescribed as 62.5 micrograms. 62.5 tells us that there are six 'tens', two 'ones' and five 'tenths'. *Figure 2.3* illustrates the positions of whole numbers and parts of whole numbers or decimal fractions.

MILLIONS	HUNDRED THOUSANDS	TEN THOUSANDS	THOUSANDS	HUNDREDS	TENS	ONES/UNITS	DECIMAL POINT	TENTHS	HUNDREDTHS	THOUSANDTHS
					6	2	.	5		

Figure 2.3. *Digoxin 62.5 micrograms.*

The role of zero

Within the decimal system, zeros play an important role when there are no values. If the number 702 is used as an example, '7' indicates seven hundreds, '0' indicates no tens and '2' indicates two ones. The '0' maintains the position of the other digits within the number.

When writing numbers that contain four digits or more, you will see various different formats:

- four digits – one thousand may be seen written as 1,000 (using a comma), 1 000 (using a gap) or 1000 (closed up, no gap or comma); according to the metric (SI) system, all numbers up to 9999 should be written with no space and no comma

- five or more digits – ten thousand five hundred may be seen written as 10,500, 10 500 or 10500; this book again uses the SI convention and presents all numbers above 10 000 with a space.

These standards should be used in healthcare and this approach has safety advantages because the comma cannot then be mistaken for a decimal point.

ERROR ALERT

Zeros can maintain the position of other digits, but they can also be the source of errors. When calculating and giving medications or fluids, it is critical to remove any trailing zeros – ones used after the decimal point that don't maintain the position of other digits within a number. For example, five milligrams should be written as 5 mg and not 5.0 mg. If the decimal point is not clear, the result is a ten times overdose.

Self-assessment test 2.1: digit value

The recap questions below will help to consolidate your learning about the value of digits within a number. Answers can be found at the end of the book.

1 In the number 1.65, what value does the digit '5' have?

2 In the number 6.079, what value does the digit '0' have?

3 In the number 8.125, what value does the digit '5' have?

4 In the number 4 012 000, what value does the digit '4' have?

Self-assessment test 2.1: digit value (*continued*)

5   In the number 12.75, what value does the digit '2' have?

6   In the number 2.09, what value does the digit '9' have?

7   In the number 725.3, what value does the digit '3' have?

8   In the number 7.005, what value does the digit '5' have?

9   In the number 0.13, what value does the digit '3' have?

10   In the number 9.125, what value does the digit '5' have?

2.3 **Addition**

Most simple additions can be performed mentally, but where many individual numbers have to be added together, like when adding up the fluid intake of a patient over twenty-four hours, the potential for error increases. In these circumstances, it is sensible to perform the calculation on paper.

The numbers are written down in a column format as in the example below. This ensures that the numbers are lined up correctly for the calculation and maintains the place value of each digit within the number. When adding two or more numbers together, the calculation can be performed in any order: 74 + 26 gives the same answer as 26 + 74.

SENSE CHECK

As well as being able to perform calculations, you need to learn ways of checking to make sure you haven't made a careless mistake. Remember that if you add numbers together, your answer must be greater than the numbers that you started with.

Use the following procedure to check your addition answers:
- take one of the numbers that you added up away from the answer
- for example, 6 + 9 = 15 and therefore 15 − 9 = 6.

EXAMPLE 2.1

The columns are not usually labelled as hundreds (H), tens (T) or ones (O), but this helps to illustrate the calculation.

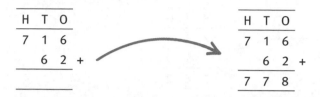

```
H  T  O          H  T  O
7  1  6          7  1  6
   6  2 +           6  2 +
                 7  7  8
```

Method
The addition is calculated vertically from right to left, starting under the 'ones' column and involves three individual calculations, one for the 'ones' column, one for the 'tens' column and a final calculation for the 'hundreds' column.

Process
Starting with the 'ones' column:
6 + 2 = 8

```
H  T  O
7  1  6
   6  2 +
      8
```

Moving left to the 'tens' column:
1 + 6 = 7

```
H  T  O
7  1  6
   6  2 +
   7  8
```

Moving left to the 'hundreds' column:
7 + 0 = 7

```
H  T  O
7  1  6
   6  2 +
7  7  8
```

This gives the answer of 7 hundreds, 7 tens and 8 ones, or 778.

Checking
To check your answer: 778 − 62 = 716.

Not all additions are this straightforward as there will be times when the calculation results in ten or more in a column, such as in *Example 2.2*.

EXAMPLE 2.2

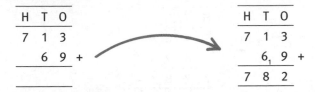

```
H  T  O              H  T  O
7  1  3              7  1  3
   6  9 +               6₁ 9 +
                     7  8  2
```

Method
As before, the addition is calculated vertically from right to left, starting under the 'ones' column.

Process
Starting with the 'ones' column:
  3 + 9 = 12

```
H  T  O
7  1  3
   6₁ 9 +
      2
```

• The number '12' is made up of one 'ten' and two 'ones'. Because this column is only used to record the 'ones', the two 'ones' are recorded here and the 'ten' is carried over to the 'tens' column. The usual way of doing this is to write a small '1' by the 6 under the 'tens' column.

Moving left to the 'tens' column:
  1 + 6 + 1 (carried over from the 'ones' column) = 8

```
H  T  O
7  1  3
   6₁ 9 +
   8  2
```

Moving left to the 'hundreds' column:
  7 + 0 = 7

```
H  T  O
7  1  3
   6₁ 9 +
7  8  2
```

This gives the answer of 7 hundreds, 8 tens and 2 ones, or 782.

Checking
To check your answer: 782 − 69 = 713.

EXAMPLE 2.3

Fluid balance charts are used to monitor the fluid intake and output of patients. You will need to add up fairly large numbers, particularly when monitoring urine output. If a patient passed 425 millilitres of urine after breakfast and has passed 485 millilitres just before lunch, how much urine have they passed during the morning?

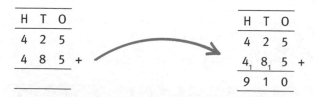

Method
Perform the addition calculation vertically from right to left, starting under the 'ones' column.

Process
Starting with the 'ones' column:
5 + 5 = 10

H	T	O
4	2	5
4	8₁	5 +
		0

- The number '10' is made up of one 'ten' and no 'ones'. Because this column is only used to record the 'ones', a zero is recorded here and the 'ten' is carried over to the 'tens' column. The usual way of doing this is to write a small '1' by the 8 under the 'tens' column.

Moving left to the 'tens' column:
2 + 8 + 1 (carried over from the 'ones' column) = 11

H	T	O
4	2	5
4₁	8₁	5 +
	1	0

- This part of the calculation is being performed under the tens column, therefore the number '11' is made up of one 'hundred' and one 'ten' (eleven lots of ten). Because this column is only used to record 'tens', a one is recorded here and the hundred is carried over to the 'hundreds' column, identified as a small '1' by the 4 under the 'hundreds' column.

Moving left to the 'hundreds' column:
4 + 4 + 1 (carried over from the
'tens' column) = 9

H	T	O	
4	2	5	
4₁	8₁	5	+
9	1	0	

This gives the answer of 9 hundreds, 1 ten and no ones or 910. So the total amount of urine passed during the morning is 910 millilitres.

Checking
To check your answer 910 – 485 = 425.

TOP TIP

It may seem tiresome adding up large amounts of numbers but persevere and don't resort to using the calculator on your mobile phone. The standards expected of a registered nurse dictate that you must be able to perform calculations without the use of a calculator. Practice helps in the development of numeracy confidence.

Self-assessment test 2.2: addition

The recap questions below will help to consolidate your learning about additions. Answers can be found at the end of the book.

1 23 + 77 =

2 156 + 239 =

3 17 + 3294 =

4 21006 + 2005 =

5 179 + 642 =

6 130 + 150 + 190 + 250 + 80 + 225 =

7 125 + 145 + 155 + 68 + 95 + 300 =

8 500 + 200 + 150 + 45 + 60 + 120 + 397 =

9 220 + 140 + 50 + 65 + 72 + 168 =

10 85 + 33 + 120 + 235 + 128 + 50 =

Self-assessment test 2.2: addition (*continued*)

11 During the course of a morning, a patient drinks the following amounts of fluid: tea 180 millilitres, orange 100 millilitres, water 120 millilitres, milk 125 millilitres and coffee 150 millilitres. What is the total amount of fluid that the patient receives?

12 A patient has a chest drain following surgery. Over the course of 24 hours, it drains: 125 millilitres, 70 millilitres and 40 millilitres. In addition, the patient is nauseous and vomits on four occasions, losing the following amounts of fluid: 250 millilitres, 150 millilitres, 120 millilitres and 90 millilitres. What is the total amount of fluid lost over the 24-hour period?

2.4 Subtraction

Subtractions involve taking one number away from another. In the clinical environment they are used in the calculation of fluid balance records to determine if the patient is in a negative or positive state of fluid balance and they are also used to calculate the stock levels of controlled drugs following administration.

The same basic rules apply as they did for additions. It is important that the digit positions are maintained to avoid errors and this is where the use of columns can help. Usually, but this is not always the case, a smaller number is taken away from a larger number, so place the larger number at the top and the smaller number below it. When calculating fluid balance records, for example, the fluid loss from the body can be greater than the input and so in this case you are calculating the difference between the input (this number at the top) and the output (this number at the bottom). *Chapter 5* covers this in more detail.

SENSE CHECK

Don't forget to check that you haven't made a basic error with your calculation. If you subtract, the answer must be less than the number that you started with.

Use the following procedure to check your subtraction answers:
- add your answer to the number that you took away
- for example 34 − 22 = 12 so therefore 12 + 22 = 34.

EXAMPLE 2.4

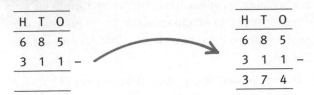

```
H  T  O          H  T  O
6  8  5          6  8  5
3  1  1  –       3  1  1  –
                 3  7  4
```

Method

The subtraction is calculated vertically from right to left, starting under the 'ones' column and involves three individual calculations, one for the 'ones' column, one for the 'tens' column and a final calculation for the 'hundreds' column.

Process

Starting with the 'ones' column:

5 – 1 = 4

```
H  T  O
6  8  5
3  1  1  –
      4
```

Moving left to the 'tens' column:

8 – 1 = 7

```
H  T  O
6  8  5
3  1  1  –
   7  4
```

Moving left to the 'hundreds' column:

6 – 3 = 3

```
H  T  O
6  8  5
3  1  1  –
3  7  4
```

This gives the answer of 3 hundreds, 7 tens and 4 ones, or 374.

Checking

To check your answer: 374 + 311 = 685.

Not all subtractions are straightforward because there will be times when the calculation requires you to take a larger number from a smaller number; see *Example 2.5* in which you need to take 5 from 3.

EXAMPLE 2.5

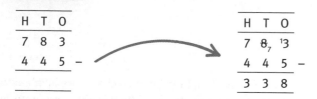

```
H  T  O          H  T  O
7  8  3          7  8₇ ¹3
4  4  5  –       4  4  5  –
                 3  3  8
```

Method

As before, the subtraction is calculated vertically from right to left, starting under the 'ones' column.

Process

Starting with the 'ones' column:

$5 - 3 =$

- You cannot take 5 from 3 because 3 is less than 5. The way around this is to borrow 1 'ten' from the 8 'tens' under the 'ten' column. When this is transferred to the 'ones' column, this is added to the 3 to give 13. The usual way of doing this is to write a small '1' by the 3 under the 'ones' column. The 8 under the 'tens' column needs to be reduced to 7 to account for 1 ten being borrowed by the 'ones' column. This involves crossing out the 8 and replacing it with a 7.

The subtraction now becomes:

$13 - 5 = 8$

```
H  T  O
7  8₇ ¹3
4  4  5  –
      8
```

Moving left to the 'tens' column:

$7 - 4 = 3$

```
H  T  O
7  8₇ ¹3
4  4  5  –
   3  8
```

Moving left to the 'hundreds' column:

$7 - 4 = 3$

```
H  T  O
7  8₇ ¹3
4  4  5  –
3  3  8
```

This gives the answer of 3 hundreds, 3 tens and 8 ones, or 338.

Checking
To check your answer: 338 + 445 = 783.

EXAMPLE 2.6

When monitoring a patient's state of hydration, fluid balance charts are invaluable. These involve calculating the amount of various types of fluid input and output as well as the total input and output from the body.

The overall fluid balance is calculated by subtracting the output from the input. If a patient's total input over 24 hours was 2455 millilitres and their output was 2260 millilitres, you can calculate their fluid balance as follows.

```
Th  H  T  O              Th  H  T  O
 2  4  5  5               2  4₃ ¹5 5
 2  2  6  0  –            2  2  6  0  –
                          _____
                             1  9  5
```

Method
As before, the subtraction is calculated vertically from right to left, starting under the 'ones' column. Note that an additional column for 'thousands' has been included because the numbers are in the thousands.

Process
Starting with the 'ones' column:
  5 – 0 = 5

```
Th  H  T  O
 2  4  5  5
 2  2  6  0  –
_____
             5
```

Moving left to the 'tens' column:
  5 – 6 =
- You cannot take 6 from 5, because it is a lower number. The way around this is to borrow 1 'hundred' from the 4 'hundreds' under the 'hundreds' column. When this is transferred to the 'tens' column, this is added to the 5 to give 15. This is recorded by writing a small '1' by the 5 under the 'tens' column. The 4 under the 'hundreds' column needs to be reduced to 3 to account for 1 hundred being borrowed by the 'tens' column. This involves crossing out the 4 and replacing it with a 3.

The subtraction now becomes:
15 − 6 = 9

Th	H	T	O
2	4₃	¹5	5
2	2	6	0 −
		9	5

Moving left to the 'hundreds' column:
3 − 2 = 1

Th	H	T	O
2	4₃	¹5	5
2	2	6	0 −
	1	9	5

Moving left to the 'thousands' column:
2 − 2 = 0

Th	H	T	O
2	4₃	¹5	5
2	2	6	0 −
	1	9	5

This gives the answer of 0 thousands, 1 hundred, 9 tens and 5 ones, or 195. Therefore the patient's input was 195 millilitres more than their output.

Checking
To check your answer: 195 + 2260 = 2455.

Self-assessment test 2.3: subtraction

The recap questions below will help to consolidate your learning about subtractions. Answers can be found at the end of the book.

1   155 − 42 =

2   1276 − 165 =

3   916 − 817 =

4   96 − 58 =

5   117 − 99 =

6   2139 − 126 =

Self-assessment test 2.3: subtraction (*continued*)

7 6483 – 5261 =

8 2912 – 1915 =

9 792 – 689 =

10 542 – 454 =

11 If a patient's total fluid input over 24 hours was 3205 millilitres and their output was 2410 millilitres, what is their overall fluid balance?

12 A patient takes morphine sulphate solution 10 mg in 5 millilitres orally, six times each day. The ward stock bottle contains 250 millilitres. How much will be left in the bottle after seven days?

2.5 Multiplication

Multiplication is the same as repeatedly adding the same number together, for example, 5 × 12 is the same as 12 + 12 + 12 + 12 + 12, but the process is less time consuming. Multiplications are used to calculate fluid balance charts where the same volume has been given repeatedly and when calculating drug doses that are prescribed per kilogram of body weight.

Many people remember their 'times tables' from school. If you didn't learn these or have forgotten them, you might find that a copy of the 'multiplication grid' in *Appendix 5* acts as a valuable resource. If you don't know your times tables, it's worth practising them until you are confident that you can do simple multiplications in your head.

When multiplying two or more numbers together, the calculation can be performed in any order, so 25 × 4 gives the same answer as 4 × 25.

To check your multiplications

Divide your answer by one of the numbers you multiplied.

For example 6 × 4 = 24 therefore 24 ÷ 4 = 6.

EXAMPLE 2.7

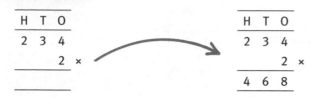

```
H  T  O              H  T  O
2  3  4              2  3  4
      2 ×                  2 ×
                     4  6  8
```

Method

The multiplication is calculated vertically from right to left, starting under the 'ones' column and involves three individual calculations, one for the 'ones' column, one for the 'tens' column and a final calculation for the 'hundreds' column.

Process

Starting with the 'ones' column:

$2 \times 4 = 8$

```
H  T  O
2  3  4
      2 ×
      8
```

Moving left to the 'tens' column:

$2 \times 3 = 6$

```
H  T  O
2  3  4
      2 ×
   6  8
```

Moving left to the 'hundreds' column:

$2 \times 2 = 4$

```
H  T  O
2  3  4
      2 ×
4  6  8
```

This gives the answer of 4 hundreds, 6 tens and 8 ones, or 468.

Checking

To check your answer: $468 \div 2 = 234$.

Not all multiplications are as straightforward as this. There will be times when the calculation results in ten or more in a column, such as in *Example 2.8*.

EXAMPLE 2.8

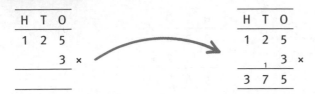

> **Method**
> As before, the multiplication is calculated vertically from right to left, starting under the 'ones' column and involves three individual calculations, one for the 'ones' column, one for the 'tens' column and a final calculation for the 'hundreds' column.

Process

Starting with the 'ones' column:
    $3 \times 5 = 15$

H	T	O
1	2	5
	₁	3 ×
		5

• The number '15' is made up of one 'ten' and five 'ones'. Because this column is only used to record the 'ones', the five 'ones' are recorded here and the 'ten' carried over to the 'tens' column. The usual way of doing this is to write a small '1' below the 2 under the 'tens' column.

Moving left to the 'tens' column:
    $3 \times 2 = 6$ plus the 1 which was carried over from the 'ones' column = 7

H	T	O
1	2	5
	₁	3 ×
	7	5

Moving left to the 'hundreds' column:
    $3 \times 1 = 3$

H	T	O
1	2	5
	₁	3 ×
3	7	5

This gives the answer of 3 hundreds, 7 tens and 5 ones, or 375.

> **Checking**
> To check your answer: $375 \div 3 = 125$.

This process works well when the multiplication involves one number that is less than ten. When both of the numbers to be multiplied together are greater than ten, an extra stage of calculation is necessary.

EXAMPLE 2.9

A fluid balance chart shows that a patient's oral intake in one 24-hour period was 11 glasses of water. Each glass measures 85 ml. What is the total oral intake? This calculation involves multiplying 85 and 11.

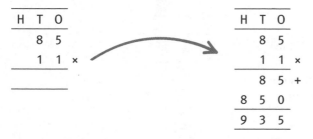

H	T	O
	8	5
	1	1 ×

H	T	O
	8	5
	1	1 ×
	8	5 +
8	5	0
9	3	5

Method
As before, the multiplication is calculated vertically from right to left, making sure that individual digits are kept in position within the columns. The terms 'ones', 'tens' or 'hundreds' column used within the explanation only refer to the top number in the calculation.

Process
The multiplication has two stages, firstly multiplying the top number by the 1 'one' belonging to the 11 and secondly multiplying the top number by the 1 'ten' belonging to the 11.

Stage one
Starting with the 'ones' column:
    1 × 5 = 5

H	T	O
	8	5
	1	1 ×
		5

Moving left to the 'tens' column:
    1 × 8 = 8

H	T	O
	8	5
	1	1 ×
	8	5

Stage two

Stage two starts by placing a 'zero' under the 'ones' column to maintain the place of the other digits. This is done because the number being used in the multiplication from the bottom line is a ten, not a 'one'.

H	T	O	
	8	5	
	1	1	×
	8	5	+
		0	

Starting with the 'ones' column:
$1 \times 5 = 5$
but the answer is put under the 'tens' column because this is really $10 \times 5 = 50$.

H	T	O	
	8	5	
	1	1	×
	8	5	+
	5	0	

Moving left to the 'tens' column:
$1 \times 8 = 8$
but the answer is recorded under the 'hundreds' column because this is really $10 \times 80 = 800$.

H	T	O	
	8	5	
	1	1	×
	8	5	+
8	5	0	

The results of the two separate multiplications are then added together:

H	T	O	
	8	5	
	1	1	×
	8	5	+
8	5	0	
9	3	5	

So the total oral intake of fluid over the 24-hour period is 935 ml.

Checking
To check your answer: $935 \div 11 = 85$.

TOP TIP

Remember that:
- an even number multiplied by an even number always makes an even number
- an even number multiplied by an odd number always makes an even number
- an odd number multiplied by an odd number always makes an odd number.

Self-assessment test 2.4: multiplication

The recap questions below will help to consolidate your learning about multiplications. Answers can be found at the end of the book.

1 $15 \times 4 =$

2 $23 \times 6 =$

3 $35 \times 9 =$

4 $26 \times 22 =$

5 $72 \times 18 =$

6 $124 \times 12 =$

7 $161 \times 13 =$

8 $148 \times 17 =$

9 $257 \times 14 =$

10 $321 \times 67 =$

11 You need to order an inhaler to last a patient for the next 28 days. The patient takes four inhalations (doses) of the inhaler daily. How many inhalations does the patient take over 28 days and will an inhaler containing 200 doses be sufficient for that period?

12 A patient is due to go home for the weekend. They take 5 millilitres of an oral solution four times each day. Over the weekend they will need: one dose for Friday night, four doses for Saturday, four doses for Sunday and one dose for Monday morning. How many millilitres need to be in the bottle to last until the patient returns to hospital?

Multiplying decimals

Clinical calculations will sometimes involve multiplying decimals together. Treat this as you would any other multiplication and then use the technique below to get the decimal point in exactly the right place.

Imagine that you had to calculate the annual leave entitlement for a member of staff. Nurse Williams is a Practice nurse and is entitled to 2.33 days annual leave for each month that she works. She has worked at the surgery for 4.5 months. How much time off is she owed?

To calculate the amount of annual leave that she can take means multiplying 2.33 (days) by 4.5 (months):

H	T	O	t	h	
		2.	3	3	
		4.	5		×

H	T	O	t	h	
		2.	3	3	
		4.	5		×
	1	1,	6,	5	
	9,	3,	2	0	
1	,0	4	8	5	

> **Method**
> As before, the multiplication is calculated vertically from right to left, starting under the 'hundredths' column (h) and involves three individual calculations, one for the 'hundredths' column (h), one for the 'tenths' (t) column and a final calculation for the 'ones' column. The results of these three individual calculations are then added together.

Process
Starting with the bottom number at the 'tenths' column:
The digit 5 from the number 4.5 is used to multiply the digit 3 in the 'hundredths' column from the 2.33. It is then used to multiply the digit 3 in the 'tenths' column and then the digit 2 from the number 2.33.
$5 \times 3 = 15$
- Similar to the earlier multiplication examples, the 5 from the 15 is recorded below the line beneath the hundredths column and the 1 from the 15 is carried over to the 'tenths' column (written as a small '1' in this column).

H	T	O	t	h
		2.	3	3
		4.	5	×
			1	5

The digit 5 from the number 4.5 is then used to multiply the digit 3 in the 'tenths' column from the number 2.33

5 × 3 = 15

and the 1 carried over is added

15 + 1 = 16

- The 6 'ones' in this number are written below the line beneath the 5 of the number 4.5 under the 'tenths' column and the 1 'ten' from this number is carried over to the 'ones' column

H	T	O	t	h
		2.	3	3
		4.	5	×
	1		6,₁	5

The digit 5 from the number 4.5 is then used to multiply the digit 2 in the 'ones' column from the number 2.33

5 × 2 = 10

and the 1 carried over is added

10 + 1 = 11

- The 1 'one' in this number is written below the line beneath the 4 of the number 4.5 under the 'ones' column and the 1 'ten' from this number is written below the line in the 'tens' column

H	T	O	t	h
		2.	3	3
		4.	5	×
	1	1,₁	6,₁	5

Moving left to the 'ones' column:

The first action is to write a zero in the 'hundredths' column below the 5 in the first part of the answer. The overall answer to this calculation is calculated by adding up three short answers and this zero acts as a placeholder within the short answer, maintaining the value of the digits.

H	T	O	t	h
		2.	3	3
		4.	5	×
	1	1,₁	6,₁	5
				0

The digit 4 from the number 4.5 is used to multiply the digit 3 in the 'hundredths' column from the 2.33. It is then used to multiply the digit 3 in the 'tenths' column and then the digit 2 from the number 2.33

$4 \times 3 = 12$

- Similar to the earlier multiplication examples, the 2 from the 12 is recorded below the line beneath the 'tenths' column and the 1 from the 12 is carried over to the 'ones' column (written as a small '1' in this column).

H	T	O	t	h
		2.	3	3
		4.	5		×
	1	1,	6,	5
			2	0
		1		

The digit 4 from the number 4.5 is then used to multiply the digit 3 in the 'tenths' column from the number 2.33

$4 \times 3 = 12$

and the 1 carried over is added

$12 + 1 = 13$

- The 3 'ones' in this number are written below the line beneath the 4 of the number 4.5 under the 'ones' column and the 1 'ten' from this number is carried over to the 'tens' column (written as a small '1' in this column).

H	T	O	t	h
		2.	3	3
		4.	5		×
	1	1,	6,	5
		3,	2	0
	1			

The digit 4 from the number 4.5 is then used to multiply the digit 2 in the 'ones' column from the number 2.33

$4 \times 2 = 8$

and the 1 carried over is added

$8 + 1 = 9$

- This number is written below the line in the 'tens' column.

H	T	O	t	h
		2.	3	3
		4.	5		×
	1	1,	6,	5
	9,	3,	2	0

The next stage of the calculation involves adding up the individual answer numbers that are written below the original sum.

```
H  T  O  t  h
      2. 3  3
      4. 5       ×
   1  1₁ 6₁ 5
   9₁ 3₁ 2  0
1  ₁0 4  8  5
```

The final stage of the process is identifying the correct location for the decimal point. This is obtained by adding up the number of digits to the right of the decimal point in the numbers being multiplied together. The upper number 2.33 has two digits after the decimal point and the lower number 4.5 has one digit after the decimal point. Adding these together gives three digits, so there are three digits after the decimal point in the answer, making our final answer 10.485.

Checking

Checking the answer to your calculation can be done like other multiplications, by division: $10.485 \div 4.5 = 2.33$ but this is a complex division. (The nurse checking this calculation could use a calculator but the nurse performing the calculation should not.)

An alternative is to estimate the answer. This doesn't give an exact answer but guides you to the number you would expect to see the answer close to. A rough estimation of this answer involves rounding 4.5 up to 5 and 2.33 down to 2, which would give an estimate of $5 \times 2 = 10$. Remember that this estimation is to provide guidance for placing the decimal point. The alternative positions for the decimal point would result in the answer being 1.0485 or 104.85, and both of these are clearly far from the estimation.

If you're feeling confident, a more accurate estimate would be to say that 2.33 is almost exactly $2\frac{1}{3}$; 2×4.45 is close to 9, and $\frac{1}{3} \times 4.5$ is 1.5 – adding 9 and 1.5 gives 10.5.

Self-assessment test 2.5: multiplying decimals

The recap questions below will help to consolidate your learning about multiplying decimals. Answers can be found at the end of the book.

1 To help with the development of her academic work, a lecturer has agreed to provide Student Nurse Vipond with 0.75 hours of supervision each week for the next 8.5 weeks. How much supervision will she receive?

2 Student Nurse Jones has to complete an assignment over the next week. She has calculated that if she writes 2.5 pages per day for 5.5 days, she will achieve more than the minimum of 12 pages. Is she correct?

3 A patient with heart failure and fluid retention needs to lose 0.75 litres of fluid per day for the next 2.5 days. How much fluid will they lose in total?

4 A seriously ill patient is having their urine output measured hourly. They have excreted 0.06 litres of urine per hour over the last 3.5 hours. What is the total urine output over the 3.5 hours?

5 A patient is set the weight loss target of 1.25 kg per month for 2.5 months. How much weight in total should the patient lose over the 2.5 months?

6 A trauma patient has been receiving intravenous fluid at a rate of 0.25 litres of fluid per hour for the last 4.5 hours. How much intravenous fluid have they received in total?

7 A registered nurse earns £14.40 per hour. How much will she earn for 18.25 hours work?

2.6 Division

Dividing is a process that involves sharing quantities into equal parts, for example 72 divided by 6 (written as 72 ÷ 6). In this example, we want to find out how many times 6 goes into 72. There are two symbols used to indicate that the calculation is a division, ÷ or one number placed above another, separated by a line − .

$$72 \div 6 = \quad or \quad \frac{72}{6} =$$

Divisions are frequently used to calculate the hourly flow rate of intravenous fluids administered to patients. If 500 ml of an intravenous solution is prescribed over 4 hours, the calculation is 500 divided by 4.

SENSE CHECK

Use the following procedure to check your division answers:
• Multiply your answer by the number that was used to divide by.

For example $36 \div 9 = 4$ therefore $4 \times 9 = 36$

When calculating divisions, the method used is different to that used for additions, subtractions and multiplications in that the calculation starts at the left of the number.

EXAMPLE 2.10

$126 \div 3 =$

Method
The division is calculated from left to right, starting under the largest unit column, in this example 'hundreds'.

Process
Starting with the 'hundreds' column:
   3 divided into 1 ($1 \div 3$) will not
   go because 1 is smaller than 3.
   So 3 is divided into 12 ($12 \div 3 = 4$),
   placing the 4 above the line
   in the 'tens' column.

$$\begin{array}{c c c} H & T & O \\ \hline & 4 & \\ 3 \overline{)\,1} & 2 & 6 \end{array}$$

3 is now divided into the remaining
6 ($6 \div 3 = 2$) and the result placed
above in the 'ones' column.

$$\begin{array}{c c c} H & T & O \\ \hline & 4 & 2 \\ 3 \overline{)\,1} & 2 & 6 \end{array}$$

This gives the answer of 4 'tens' and 2 'ones' or 42.

Checking
To check your answer: $3 \times 42 = 126$

> **ERROR ALERT**
>
> A patient receiving treatment for breathing problems in a Merseyside hospital died suddenly and unexpectedly. The dose of aminophylline (a drug used to relax the airways and improve breathing) intended to be infused over 24 hours was given in 20 minutes. This might look like an error made when calculating a division, because this can be used to work out the hourly rate of infusion. However, in this case, the drug was being infused by an electronic device that performed the calculation. It is probable that human error when inputting the volumes and time of infusion caused this tragic event.

EXAMPLE 2.11

A patient needs to receive 68 milligrams of a drug in four doses. How many milligrams will be in each dose? The calculation is 68 ÷ 4.

> **Method**
> The division is calculated from left to right, starting under the largest unit column, in this example 'tens'.

Process

Starting with the 'tens' column:
    4 divided into 6 (6 ÷ 4) goes once.
    To record this, a 1 is written above
    the line in the 'tens' column.

$$
\begin{array}{c|c|c}
H & T & O \\
\hline
 & 1 & \\
\hline
4\overline{)} & 6 & 8
\end{array}
$$

Because 4 does not divide into 6 exactly, we need to find out what remains.

Finding the remainder:
    This is done by subtracting 4 from 6 (6 − 4) which equals 2 and recording this as a small number to the left of the number in the 'ones' column, to make 28. This procedure is done every time a number doesn't divide exactly into another one.

$$
\begin{array}{c|c|c}
H & T & O \\
\hline
 & 1 & \\
\hline
4\overline{)} & 6 & {}^2 8
\end{array}
$$

Completing the division:
    4 is then divided into the number(s) in the 'ones' column; here this is the remainder 2 from the 'tens' column and the original 8 from the 'ones' column to make the number 28.

4 is divided into 28 (28 ÷ 4) and the result 7 is placed above the line in the 'ones' column. As 28 ÷ 4 = 7 exactly, there is no need to find a remainder.

```
      H   T   O
              
          1   7
  4 )     6  ²8
```

This gives the answer of 1 'ten' and 7 'ones' or 17, so there are 17 milligrams in each of the four doses.

Checking
To check your answer: 17 × 4 = 68.

Self-assessment test 2.6: division

The recap questions below will help to consolidate your learning about divisions. Answers can be found at the end of the book.

1 49 ÷ 7 =

2 84 ÷ 8 =

3 117 ÷ 9 =

4 72 ÷ 6 =

5 51 ÷ 4 =

6 87.5 ÷ 7 =

7 172 ÷ 8 =

8 67.5 ÷ 4 =

9 45 ÷ 6 =

10 130.5 ÷ 9 =

11 Over 8 hours a patient needs to receive 840 millilitres of intravenous fluid. How many millilitres need to be given each hour?

12 A syringe driver contains medication diluted in 96 millilitres of fluid. It is programmed to inject the medication at 16 millilitres per hour. How many hours will it take to administer the medication?

Long division

Some divisions are more complex such as the one in *Example 2.12* below and in these cases a modified method can be used.

EXAMPLE 2.12

$221 \div 13 =$

Method
The division is calculated from left to right, starting under the largest unit column – 'hundreds'.

Process
Starting with the 'hundreds' column:
   13 divided into 2 (2 ÷ 13) will not go because 2 is smaller than 13. 13 is now divided into 22 (22 ÷ 13) which goes once. To record this, a 1 is written above the line in the 'tens' column.

```
        H   T   O
            1
  13)   2   2   1
```

As 13 does not divide into 22 exactly, we need to find out what remains.

Finding the remainder:
   This is done by subtracting 13 from 22 (22 – 13) which equals 9. In *Example 2.11* above we placed this remainder number next to the number in the 'ones' and then carried on the division in the same way. However, for more complex divisions it can be useful to record each stage of the calculation as follows:
* Start by writing the 13 underneath the 22 and then subtract 13 from 22 to give 9
* Record the 9 below the 3 in the 'tens' column
* This procedure is done every time a number doesn't divide exactly into another one.

```
        H   T   O
            1   7
    13) 2   2   1
        1   3
            9
```

Completing the division:

13 is then divided into the remainder 9 (9 ÷ 13) but this won't go because 13 is larger than 9 so the 1 from the 'ones' column of 221 is brought down to make this number 91.

13 can then be divided into 91 (91 ÷ 13) and the result 7 is placed above the line in the 'ones' column. As 91 ÷ 13 = 7 exactly, there is no need to find a remainder.

```
        H   T │ O
            1 │ 7
    13) 2   2 │ 1
        1   3 │ ↓
            9 │ 1
```

Answer:

This gives the answer of 1 'ten' and 7 'ones' or 17.

Checking

To check your answer: 17 × 13 = 221.

TOP TIP

In some divisions, you can use the multiplication grid to identify how many times a number goes into another. For example 72 ÷ 9 = 8 because the grid tells us that 8 × 9 = 72.

If like in *Example 2.12*, the number isn't on the multiplication grid, create your own:

1 × 13 = 13
2 × 13 = 26
3 × 13 = 39
4 × 13 = 52
5 × 13 = 65
6 × 13 = 78
7 × 13 = 91

EXAMPLE 2.13

In 26 millilitres of an oral solution, there are 650 milligrams of a drug. How many milligrams are in each millilitre?

The calculation required is:

$650 \div 26$

Method

The division is calculated from left to right, starting under the largest unit column – 'hundreds'.

Process

Starting with the 'hundreds' column:

26 divided into 6 ($6 \div 26$) will not go because 6 is smaller than 26, so we can now use the 'hundreds' and 'tens' columns together:

26 is now divided into 65 ($65 \div 26$) which goes twice. To record this, a 2 is written above the line in the 'tens' column.

```
        H  T  O
           2
     26) 6  5  0
```

Because 26 does not divide into 65 exactly, we need to find out what remains.

Finding the remainder:

This is done by subtracting 52 (= 2 × 26) from 65 (65 – 52) which equals 1 'ten' and 3 'ones' and recording this below the 65 and 52. This procedure is done every time a number doesn't divide exactly into another one.

```
        H  T  O
           2
     26) 6  5  0
         5  2
         1  3
```

Completing the division:

26 is then divided into the remainder 13 ($26 \div 13$) but this won't go because 26 is larger than 13 so the 0 from the 'ones' column of 650 is brought down to make this number 130.

26 can then be divided into 130 ($130 \div 26$) and the result 5 is placed above the line in the 'ones' column. As $130 \div 26 = 5$ exactly, there is no need to find a remainder.

```
        H  T  O
           2
    26) 6  5  0
        5  2  ↓
        1  3  0
```

Answer:
There are 25 milligrams in each millilitre of the oral solution.

Checking
To check your answer: 25 × 26 = 650.

Long division with decimals

Divisions that involve decimals can look daunting but applying a couple of basic steps simplifies the calculation.

EXAMPLE 2.14

978.75 ÷ 13.5

Method
Faced with a calculation like this, the first thing to do is simplify the numbers. Make the number you are dividing with into a whole number by moving the decimal point to the right. In this example making 13.5 into the whole number 135 involves moving the decimal point once to the right.
Now move the decimal point in the number you are dividing into to the right, the same number of places as for the number you are dividing with. In this example, move the decimal point in 978.75 once to the right to make 9787.5
Note that this is the same as multiplying both numbers by ten. 978.75 ÷ 13.5 gives the same result as 9787.5 ÷ 135

```
        Th  H  T  O .  t

    135) 9  7  8  7.  5
```

Then continue with the usual method of long division by calculating from left to right, starting under the largest unit column, which is now 'thousands'.

Process

Starting with the 'thousands' column:

135 divided into 9 (9 ÷ 135) will not go because 9 is smaller than 135, so we use the 'thousands' and 'hundreds' columns together.

Using the 'thousands' and 'hundreds':

135 divided into 97 (97 ÷ 135) will not go as 97 is smaller than 135, so we use the 'thousands', 'hundreds' and 'tens' columns together.

Using the 'thousands', 'hundreds' and 'tens' columns:

135 is now divided into 978 (978 ÷ 135) which goes 7 times. To record this, a 7 is written above the line in the 'tens' column.

```
      Th  H  T  O  t
                7
  135) 9  7  8  7. 5
```

Because 135 does not divide exactly into 978, the remainder needs to be calculated. Finding the remainder is done the usual way, by subtracting 945 (7 × 135) from 978 (978 – 945), which equals 33.

```
      Th  H  T  O  t
                7
  135) 9  7  8  7. 5
       9  4  5
             3  3
```

The 7 from the 'ones' column is brought down to the remainder 33 to make 337. 135 is then divided into this (337 ÷ 135) which equals 2 and this is recorded above the line adjacent to the 7 from the first part of the calculation.

```
      Th  H  T  O  t
                7  2
  135) 9  7  8  7. 5
       9  4  5  ↓
             3  3  7
```

As 135 does not divide exactly into 337, again finding the remainder is necessary by subtracting 270 (2 × 135) from 337 (337 – 270) which leaves 67.

```
      Th  H   T   O    t
                  7   2
  135) 9   7   8   7.  5
      9   4   5   ↓
          3   3   7
          2   7   0
              6   7
```

As the next number (the 5 in 'tenths' column) is from beyond the decimal point, a decimal point is recorded above the line next to the 2 from the first part of the calculation.

```
      Th  H   T   O    t
                  7   2.
  135) 9   7   8   7.  5
      9   4   5   ↓
          3   3   7
          2   7   0
              6   7
```

135 does not divide into 67, so the 5 from the 'tenths' column is brought down to make 675 and 135 is divided into it (675 ÷ 135). This divides exactly 5 times and this is recorded above the line after the 7 and 2 from the earlier stages of the calculation.

```
      Th  H   T   O    t
                  7   2.  5
  135) 9   7   8   7.  5
      9   4   5   ↓
          3   3   7
          2   7   0   ↓
              6   7   5
```

Answer:
This gives an answer of 7 tens, 2 ones and 5 tenths, which is 72.5.

> **TOP TIP**
>
> Don't resort to using a calculator for the more complex calculations that you come across. As a registered nurse or midwife, you will have to be able to perform calculations manually so take advantage of this opportunity to practise.

Self-assessment test 2.7: long division

The recap questions below will help to consolidate your learning about divisions. Answers can be found at the end of the book.

1 $846 \div 16 =$

2 $630 \div 15 =$

3 $1440 \div 12 =$

4 $702 \div 36 =$

5 $465.6 \div 24 =$

6 $188.1 \div 16 =$

7 $1062.2 \div 47 =$

8 $719.2 \div 62 =$

9 $1093.75 \div 17.5 =$

10 $1163.75 \div 19 =$

11 On a trauma ward, four patients take a total of 16 co-codamol (8 mg / 500 mg) tablets between them daily. The ward stock bottle contains 192 tablets. How many days will the supply last?

12 On an oncology ward, thirteen fentanyl patches are used each day. How many days will the stock of 182 patches last for?

TOP TIP

If the calculation you are faced with involves more than one arithmetic sign (addition, subtraction, multiplication or division), there is a correct sequence to follow. Multiplication and division are of equal rank and they are performed from left to right and before addition and subtraction. Addition and subtraction are also of equal rank to each other and are performed from left to right but after multiplication and division. If the calculation includes brackets, do the calculation in the brackets first. A way of remembering the sequence is BoDMAS: **B**rackets, **o**thers, **D**ivision, **M**ultiplication, **A**ddition and **S**ubtraction.

In nursing and healthcare, you are unlikely to come across many calculations that need the BoDMAS sequence.

Calculating the ward stock of drugs to find out if there is sufficient for the next day is an example of where this could be used. If you had a stock of 80 tablets and four patients took eight per day, this can be written as:

$80 - (4 \times 8) =$

If you have another two patients taking six tablets per day, the calculation can be written as:

$80 - (4 \times 8) - (2 \times 6) =$

Using the BoDMAS sequence, the calculations in **B**rackets are performed first so the equation becomes:

$80 - 32 - 12 =$

The next stage of the sequence is **o**thers. This means other procedures like calculating powers / exponential numbers. There aren't any to perform in this calculation so move onto **D**ivision. There are no divisions to perform so we can proceed to **M**ultiplications. The only multiplications were within the brackets and these have already been performed. There are no **A**dditions (remember, all the patients are 'taking' the tablets).

The **S**ubtractions are performed from left to right:

$80 - 32 = 48$

$48 - 12 = 36$

So there will be enough tablets for the next day and 36 left over.

ERROR ALERT

Some drugs have a number in their name, for example 6-mercaptopurine. Errors have occurred because staff have confused the number with the dose or strength of the drug. Numbers used in the name of a drug do not influence the dosage.

2.7 Factors

When calculating using multiplication or division, you might have noticed patterns in the numbers. For example, the number 18 can be broken down into smaller numbers that divide into it:

- 1 and 18
- 2 and 9
- 3 and 6

These are all factors of 18.

In the same way, 32 can be broken down into factors that can be multiplied together to make 32.

Factors of 32 include:

- 1 and 32
- 2 and 16
- 4 and 8

When calculating, try to identify factors of numbers. This will help you to see patterns and relationships in numbers and assist in the development of your multiplication and division skills.

2.8 Fractions

Fractions, like decimals (see *Section 2.2*) can be used to express quantities less than one. They are part of our daily language, for example half (½) an hour or three-quarters (¾) of a mile. In the clinical environment amounts less than one should be expressed using the decimal system, for example 2.5 milligrams instead of 2½ milligrams and 1.5 litres, not 1½ litres. Fractions are still referred to in an informal manner; having half an hour for lunch is more appropriate than 0.5 hours.

Fractions like ½, meaning one of two equal parts, are termed proper fractions and are the type of fractions that nurses are most likely to see. The most common fractions used in healthcare are:

- ¼ – one-quarter

- ½ – half

- ¾ – three-quarters

- ⅓ – one-third

- ⅔ – two-thirds.

Proper fractions can be identified by the number above the line, which is called the numerator, being smaller than the number below the line, known as the denominator. The numerator tells you how many of each part there are, the denominator indicates the number of parts that make up a whole.

- The fraction ¼ means that the whole one is divided into four equal parts, but you only have one of these parts. This is displayed visually as:

A quarter can be calculated by dividing one by four (1 ÷ 4), which equals 0.25.

0.25 is a decimal fraction.

- The fraction ½ means that the whole one is divided into two equal parts, but you only have one part. This is displayed visually as:

A half can be calculated by dividing one by two (1 ÷ 2), which equals 0.5

- The fraction ¾ means that the whole one is divided into four equal parts, but you only have three parts. This is displayed visually as:

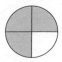

Three-quarters can be calculated by dividing one by four and then multiplying this by three (($1 \div 4$) × 3), which equals 0.75

- The fraction ⅓ means that the whole one is divided into three equal parts, but you only have one part. This is displayed visually as:

One-third can be calculated by dividing one by three ($1 \div 3$), which equals 0.33 (recurring).

- The fraction ⅔ means that the whole one is divided into three equal parts, but you only have two parts. This is displayed visually as:

Two-thirds can be calculated by dividing one by three and multiplying this by 2 (($1 \div 3$) × 2), which equals 0.66 (recurring).

In the unlikely event that you are faced with having to perform a calculation using fractions, convert them into decimal fractions as shown above. This is safer because you are less likely to make a calculation error.

2.9 Percentages

In supermarkets we are frequently offered 50% extra for the same price, as drivers we may be tempted by 10% off car insurance if we buy online, and the inflation rate is all too familiar from the news. All of these are expressed as percentages. The meaning of 'per cent' is per hundred and it is indicated by the symbol %.

Using the supermarket example, if we normally pay 99 pence for a 500 g bag of rice and the offer is for 50% extra free, we would expect to buy 750 g for 99 pence. Because 50% means 50 per hundred, in this offer for every 100 g we get 50 g free. We are buying 5 lots of 100 g, so we get 5 × 50 g free, which is 250 g extra.

An offer of 10% off car insurance means that for every £100 we spend, we receive a reduction of £10, 10% means 10 per hundred. It doesn't sound a large amount but if your insurance is normally £500 you would expect to have a reduction of £50.

The Retail Price Index (RPI) is quoted every month as a percentage and shows the price increase of selected everyday products over the past year (the inflation rate). The RPI in August 2019 was 2.8%. This means that for every £100 spent in August 2018, one year later we had to spend £102.80 to buy the same goods.

An understanding of percentages and how to calculate them is essential in clinical practice. Percentages are used:

- To express the extent of injury in patients who have sustained burns. The amount of body surface affected is estimated and is quoted as a percentage of the total body surface area. Estimation is guided by 'the rule of nines' where the arm equals 9% (of the body surface area), the head and neck equal 9%, one leg equals 18% and so on. The burn victim's palm is estimated to equal 1% of their body surface area and can be used to estimate the surface area of smaller burns.

- To indicate the strength of some medicines such as hydrocortisone cream. This is a steroid-based cream used in inflammatory skin conditions like eczema and dermatitis, and is available in strengths of 0.1%, 0.5% and 1%. The greater the percentage, the stronger the cream.

- In the routine respiratory observation of oxygen saturation levels (SaO_2). This is a simple, non-invasive technique that measures the amount of haemoglobin saturated with oxygen and is quoted as a percentage, the normal range being 93–98%.

EXAMPLE 2.15

The asthma clinic sees 75 male and 125 female patients during March. What percentage of the patients are female?

Method
Percentages are calculated by dividing the number of items in the category by the total number in the group, and then multiplying this by 100.

Process
The total number of patients is 75 + 125 = 200
The percentage of females is calculated by dividing the number of female patients by the total number of patients, then multiplying by 100:

$$\text{Females} = \frac{125}{200} \times 100 = 62.5\%$$

EXAMPLE 2.16

An acute admission unit has 25 beds, which means that during November there is a total of 750 bed days available for patient use. The unit has only used 650 of these bed days. What percentage of the bed days have been used?

Method
The total number of bed days is 750 (25 beds × 30 days in November). The number of bed days used is 650. We want to know what percentage of the total number of bed days were used.

Process
The number of bed days used is calculated by dividing the number of bed days used by the total number of bed days available, then multiplying by 100:

$$\text{Bed days used} = \frac{650}{750} \times 100 = 86.66\%$$

(This is a recurring number and can be rounded to 86.67%.)

Sometimes it is necessary to calculate a percentage change. This is useful in reflecting a numerical difference that has taken place in a situation.

The following equation can be used to calculate the percentage change:

% change = increase (or decrease) divided by the original number multiplied by 100

EXAMPLE 2.17

In the first operational year, a urology day unit treats 4240 patients. In the second year 4680 are treated. What is the percentage change in the number of patients treated?

Process
To calculate the increase (or decrease) in patient activity, subtract the original number from the new number:

4680 − 4240 = 440

To calculate the percentage change, use the equation:

(increase ÷ original number) × 100

In the urology unit example this is: (440 ÷ 4240) × 100 = 10.377%

Self-assessment test 2.8: percentages

The recap questions below will help to consolidate your learning about percentages. Answers can be found at the end of the book.

1 A local community hospital has 45 patients. There are 36 females and 9 males. What percentage of the patients are female?

2 Over a 12-month period, 50 150 patients attend an Emergency Department, 10 030 of these are children. What percentage of the patients are children?

3 A care home has 56 residents, 42 females and 14 males. What percentage of the residents are males?

4 A leg ulcer clinic has 72 registered patients with venous, arterial or ulcers of mixed causes. If 61 have venous ulcers and 4 are of mixed causes, what percentage are arterial ulcers?

5 An ophthalmic unit performed cataract procedures on 245 patients over the course of one month. 180 of the patients needed hospital transport to attend for surgery. What percentage of the patients did not require hospital transport?

6 Of 496 patients attending for surgical procedures over a period of one month, 327 required aftercare from a Community or Practice nurse. What percentage did not need aftercare?

7 A retinal screening unit invited 326 patients to attend for checks but only 287 attended. What percentage of the patients did not attend for screening?

8 An audit of surgical wound repair found that 144 patients had clips and 56 were sutured. What percentage of the patients had sutures?

9 A 40-year-old man has a resting pulse rate of 72 beats per minute. Immediately after exercise, his pulse is 104 beats per minute. What is the percentage increase in his pulse rate?

10 A 30-year-old female with asthma has a peak expiratory flow rate of 400 L/min before using her inhaler. After inhaler use, this increases to 460 L/min. What is the percentage increase in her peak expiratory flow rate?

2.10 **Ratios**

Sometimes it is necessary to provide a value that quantifies the relationship between two items or makes a numerical comparison between them. This is called a ratio. In healthcare, ratios are used to express the number of nurses in relation to the number of patients and the strength of a drug in a solution. The drug adrenaline (epinephrine in the US) used in the treatment of anaphylaxis and cardiac arrest is available in several strengths, which are expressed in ratio form. Adrenaline is available in 1 millilitre ampoules with a ratio of 1 in 1000, and 10 millilitre ampoules at 1 in 10000. When related to drugs, the first number represents weight in grams and the second number represents volume in millilitres.

Adrenaline (1 in 1000)

GRAMS (g) OR MILLIGRAMS (mg)		MILLILITRES (ml)	MILLIGRAMS PER MILLILITRES
1 g or 1000 mg	in	1000 ml	1 mg/ml

Adrenaline (1 in 10 000)

GRAMS (g) OR MILLIGRAMS (mg)		MILLILITRES (ml)	MILLIGRAMS PER MILLILITRES
1 g or 1000 mg	in	10000 ml	0.1 mg/ml

Taking staffing levels as another example, evidence indicates that there is increased risk of harm associated with a registered nurse caring for more than eight patients during a day shift. This can be expressed as a nurse-to-patient ratio of 1:8. A safer ratio would be 1:7 (or lower), while a ratio of 1:9 (or higher) could be considered a risk to patient safety.

2.11 **Expressing large numbers**

In healthcare you will sometimes see numbers written in what is known as an exponential form. An exponential or power is:

- a number that is multiplied by itself

- a way of making very large or very small numbers more manageable by reducing the number of zeros.

For example, if a laboratory report about the number of bacteria in a urine sample states that there are more than 10^4 cfu/ml ('colony forming units per millilitre of urine' – the unit of measurement used) of one micro-organism, then this can be classed as a urinary tract infection. 10^4 is the same as 10 000 which actually isn't too large to write or understand, but remember that the actual numbers of colony forming units can be much greater than this.

The number of red blood cells in a normal sample of blood is 4.5–5.4 × 10^{12} which equates to 4.5–5.4 trillion cells or 4 500 000 000 000–5 400 000 000 000 cells!

Using power forms can also reduce mistakes in the writing or reading of very large numbers.

You are most likely to see power forms used on blood results or in a physiology book indicating the normal ranges of the cellular components of blood. For example, a neutrophil (a type of white cell) count can range between 2.0 and 7.5 × 10^9 per litre. The small raised nine next to the 10 tells you that 10 is being multiplied with itself nine times, effectively telling you how many times to move the decimal point, or how many zeros to add after the one.

So 10^9 means 10 × 10 × 10 × 10 × 10 × 10 × 10 × 10 × 10 = 1 000 000 000. The neutrophil count can range from 2 × 1 000 000 000 (= 2 000 000 000) to 7.5 × 1 000 000 000 (= 7 500 000 000) per litre. In words, that would be two thousand million to seven thousand five hundred million.

PRACTICE TIP

Calculators are part of modern life and can be used by a second nurse to independently check a calculation.

Whenever possible, perform your practice calculations longhand and try using 'mental maths' to prepare yourself for your career ahead.

Self-assessment test 2.9: summary test

The recap questions below will help to consolidate your learning about the contents of this chapter; answers can be found at the end of the book.

1 In the number 84 938, what value does the digit '4' have?

2 In the number 2971.03, what value does the digit '3' have?

3 In the number 1 269 351, what value does the digit '6' have?

4 150 + 75 + 225 + 345 + 63 + 99 =

Self-assessment test 2.9: summary test (*continued*)

5 180 + 60 + 193 + 2025 + 55 + 120 + 94 =

6 220 + 30 + 960 + 710 + 1203 + 328 + 415 =

7 67 + 53 + 89 + 239 + 421 + 917 + 1501 + 27 =

8 862 − 771 =

9 1915 − 907 =

10 491 − 269 =

11 26 × 19 =

12 127 × 16 =

13 132 × 112 =

14 179 × 235 =

15 6.7 × 4.2 =

16 69.72 × 1.13 =

17 54.176 × 2.05 =

18 27.147 × 5.628 =

19 114 ÷ 8 =

20 295.2 ÷ 12 =

21 1201.2 ÷ 21 =

22 168 ÷ 19.2 =

23 Identify the factors of 24

24 Identify the factors of 39

25 Identify the factors of 66

26 Identify the factors of 82

27 Identify the factors of 90

28 Over a period of three months, 125 out of a total of 400 patients discharged from an orthopaedic unit needed an occupational therapy assessment before they could be sent home. What percentage of patients needed the assessment?

29 In a dermatology clinic, 9 out of 180 patients were unable to attend their appointment. What percentage did not attend?

30 In an audit of day surgery wound management, of 80 patient records audited only 6 experienced problems that they needed to seek further advice about. What percentage needed additional advice?

KEY POINTS TO TAKE AWAY FROM THIS CHAPTER

- Zeros play a vital role within a number, but can be a source of error if they act as trailing zeros.
- Develop ways of checking your answers and remember that calculating dosages in the healthcare environment needs estimation and numeracy skills.
- Healthcare calculations involve whole numbers and parts of numbers, decimals or fractions.

03

THE SI SYSTEM

THIS CHAPTER:

- outlines the SI units of measurement commonly used by nurses in clinical practice

- describes the units used for volume, weight and pressure and identifies the conventions of the SI system

- explains the procedure for converting within an SI unit of measurement.

3.1 Introduction

The SI system is an adaptation of the metric system and is almost universally employed in business, science and healthcare. The name SI is an abbreviation of the 'International System of Units', which was derived from the French 'Système International d'Unités'.

In healthcare, there is often a need to measure things, usually weights and volumes. In the SI system, volume is measured in litres and weight is measured in kilograms.

SI prefixes

SI units are used to quantify measurements, some extremely large and some extremely small. Standard prefixes are used to describe and name the quantities involved, irrespective of what is being measured.

The most commonly used prefixes that apply to clinical practice are:

- **Mega** – this prefix indicates millions. Benzylpenicillin, a penicillin antibiotic that is administered by injection, is available in vials containing one mega unit.

- **Milli** – this prefix indicates a thousandth of a unit. One milligram is one thousandth of a gram. Aciclovir dispersible tablets, used to treat shingles, contain 800 milligrams.

- **Micro** – this prefix indicates a millionth of a unit. One microgram is one millionth of a gram. (There are one thousand micrograms in one milligram and one thousand milligrams in one gram. One thousand multiplied by one thousand equals one million.) Glyceryl trinitrate, taken to relieve angina, is available in tablets containing 500 micrograms.

- **Nano** – this prefix indicates a thousand-millionth of a unit. This is extremely small and rarely used in clinical practice.

3.2 Volume

Volume is measured in litres or subunits of a litre, millilitres. 1000 millilitres is equal to one litre. The standard abbreviation for litre is L and the abbreviation for millilitre is ml.

Measuring volume

Drawing up medication in a syringe to accurately reflect a prescription is a common task in clinical practice. Syringes are available in several sizes. Reading the volume contained in the syringe is a prerequisite to accuracy.

SYRINGE SIZE	NUMBER OF GRADUATIONS	VOLUME OF EACH GRADUATION
1 ml	20	0.05 ml
2 ml	20	0.1 ml
5 ml	25	0.2 ml

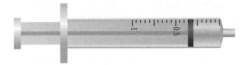

Figure 3.1. *A 1 ml syringe containing 0.3 ml.*

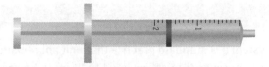

Figure 3.2. *A 2 ml syringe containing 1.6 ml.*

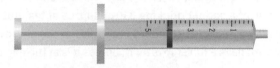

Figure 3.3. *A 5 ml syringe containing 3.8 ml.*

Some medicines such as heparin and insulin are measured in 'units'. Heparin is available in pre-loaded syringes or as a solution for injection at 5000 international units/ml or 25 000 international units/ml.

Insulin can be injected via a battery-operated pump, a pen device that uses a pre-loaded cartridge or by using a unique syringe that can measure up to 100 units. In the UK, insulin is available as U100 which means there are 100 units of insulin/ml. A prescription will state the number of units of insulin (and the type of insulin) that need to be given, for example 20 units.

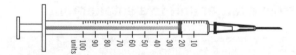

Figure 3.4. *An insulin syringe containing 20 units of insulin.*

Medicine pots are commonly used for the administration of oral solutions. When measuring liquids in a pot, read the lower meniscus line as the liquid may rise slightly against the medicine pot wall.

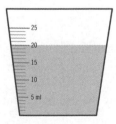

Figure 3.5. *A 25 ml medicine pot containing 20 ml.*

57

ERROR ALERT

Within the SI system it is standard practice that unit abbreviations are written in lower case, but because litre abbreviated to 'l' could be confused with the number '1', it is abbreviated to a capital letter 'L'. It is also important to remember that when expressing plurals, there is no 's' on the end of the abbreviated form. We may talk of a patient drinking 250 millilitres of tea, but when written this becomes 250 ml. It is also standard practice that the abbreviated form of the SI unit does not have a full stop after it, unless it is at the end of a sentence.

3.3 Weight

Kilograms

The SI unit of weight is the kilogram, which can be subdivided into smaller units several times. Kilograms are useful when measuring large items like body weight, but when measuring small amounts of drugs, alternative units of measurement are needed. The unit smaller than one kilogram is a gram, and 1000 grams equal one kilogram.

The abbreviation for gram is 'g'.

Converting from a larger unit to a smaller unit

RULE OF THUMB

Converting from a larger unit to a smaller unit means that you multiply by 1000.

Converting from a smaller unit to a larger unit means that you divide by 1000.

To convert 0.125 kilograms to grams:

$0.125 \times 1000 = 125$ grams

It's useful to remember that when multiplying by 1000, the decimal point moves three places to the right, i.e. one place for each zero.

0.125 becomes 125 (arrows show the decimal point move)

Converting from a smaller unit to a larger unit

To convert 125 grams to kilograms:

$125 \div 1000 = 0.125$ kg

Remember that when dividing by 1000, the decimal point moves three places to the left.

125 becomes 0.125 (arrows show the decimal point move)

Self-assessment test 3.1: converting kilograms and grams

The recap questions below will help to consolidate your learning about conversions between these two units of measurement. Answers can be found at the end of the book.

1 How many grams are in 1.3 kg?

2 How many grams are in 1.25 kg?

3 How many grams are in 0.8 kg?

4 How many grams are in 0.125 kg?

5 How many grams are in 1.204 kg?

6 How many grams are in 0.5 kg?

7 How many grams are in 2.03 kg?

8 How many grams are in 0.032 kg?

9 How many grams are in 1.005 kg?

10 How many grams are in 0.002 kg?

11 How many kg are in 2500 grams?

12 How many kg are in 4025 grams?

13 How many kg are in 750 grams?

14 Identify the amount shown on the scale:

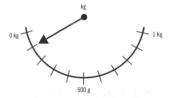

15 Identify the amount shown on the scale:

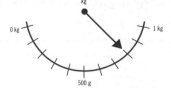

Grams and milligrams

Grams are widely used within clinical practice in drug administration. Grams can be divided into smaller units called milligrams; there are 1000 milligrams in one gram. Two 500 milligram paracetamol tablets are the equivalent of one gram. The correct abbreviation of milligram is 'mg'. Morphine is an opioid analgesic frequently used to control severe pain; it can be injected (intramuscularly, intravenously, and subcutaneously) and administered orally. As an oral solution, it is available in several different strengths. One of these contains 2 mg in 1 ml, therefore in 5 ml there are 10 mg.

Self-assessment test 3.2: converting grams and milligrams

The recap questions below will help to consolidate your learning about conversions between these two units of measurement. Answers can be found at the end of the book.

1 How many milligrams are in 1.04 g?

2 How many milligrams are in 1.005 g?

3 How many milligrams are in 0.001 g?

4 How many milligrams are in 2.202 g?

5 How many milligrams are in 1.016 g?

6 How many milligrams are in 0.33 g?

7 How many milligrams are in 0.75 g?

8 How many milligrams are in 0.06 g?

9 How many milligrams are in 1.018 g?

10 How many milligrams are in 0.106 g?

11 How many grams are in 1500 mg?

12 How many grams are in 2200 mg?

13 How many grams are in 900 mg?

14 Metformin is a drug used in diabetes. It is available in 850 mg tablets. Express this in grams.

15 Augmentin, an antibiotic, is available in 625 mg tablets. Express this in grams.

Micrograms

Milligrams can also be divided into smaller units called micrograms. There are 1000 micrograms in one milligram. Converting milligrams to micrograms follows the same rule as when converting kilograms to grams and grams to milligrams.

To convert 0.25 mg to micrograms:

0.25 × 1000 = 250 micrograms

Remember that when multiplying by 1000, the decimal point moves three places to the right, i.e. one place for each zero.

0.25 becomes 250 (arrows show the decimal point move)

Self-assessment test 3.3: converting milligrams and micrograms

The recap questions below will help to consolidate your learning about conversions between these two units of measurement. Answers can be found at the end of the book.

1 How many micrograms are in 1.25 mg?

2 How many micrograms are in 1.062 mg?

3 How many micrograms are in 0.075 mg?

4 How many micrograms are in 0.220 mg?

5 How many micrograms are in 1.028 mg?

6 How many micrograms are in 0.009 mg?

7 How many micrograms are in 0.7 mg?

8 How many micrograms are in 0.125 mg?

9 How many micrograms are in 1.5 mg?

10 How many micrograms are in 0.75 mg?

11 How many milligrams are in 1200 micrograms?

12 How many milligrams are in 800 micrograms?

13 How many milligrams are in 250 micrograms?

14 Salbutamol is a drug used in asthma by inhaler. Each inhalation is 100 micrograms. Express this in milligrams.

15 Glyceryl trinitrate is a drug used in angina. It is available in several strengths, but if a tablet (placed under the tongue) contains 0.6 mg, what is this amount expressed in micrograms?

PRACTICE TIP

Conventions for prescriptions state that drugs should be prescribed in whole amounts, not decimal fractions. A prescription for digoxin should read 125 micrograms, not 0.125 mg, so you must be able to convert between units.

KEY POINT SUMMARY

- 1000 micrograms = 1 milligram (mg)
- 1000 milligrams (mg) = 1 gram (g)
- 1000 grams (g) = 1 kilogram (kg)

3.4 **Pressure**

The commonly used unit for the measurement of blood pressure in clinical practice in the UK is millimetres of mercury, which has the abbreviation 'mmHg'. Capital letters aren't routinely used as abbreviations for units of measurement, but Hg is the international symbol for the element mercury. You will see this displayed on sphygmomanometers used to measure and record a patient's blood pressure.

There is also an SI unit for pressure called the pascal (abbreviation Pa), which is named after the French physicist and mathematician Blaise Pascal (1623–1662). The pascal is a small unit so you are more likely to see it referred to using the prefix kilo, as kilopascal (kPa). The prefix kilo means 1000, so one kPa is equal to 1000 pascals. One kPa is equal to approximately 7.5 mmHg.

NON-SI UNIT FOR PRESSURE MEASUREMENT	SI UNIT FOR PRESSURE MEASUREMENT	COMPARISON
millimetres of mercury mmHg	pascal Pa	1 kPa = 7.5 mmHg (approximately)

ERROR ALERT

Where drug doses depend on body weight, as when using low molecular weight heparin, accurately weigh the patient. Guessing or asking patients to estimate their body weight is a known source of drug error and a potentially dangerous practice (NPSA, 2010; Charani *et al.*, 2015; ISMP Canada, 2016).

The kPa is recognised as the standard unit for measuring blood gases in the UK, so you are likely to come across arterial blood gas analysis reports using kPa in intensive care and high dependency units, and on respiratory wards.

Blood for gas analysis is taken from an artery and is tested to find out the amount of oxygen and carbon dioxide contained within it. A unit of pressure like the kPa or mmHg is used to measure this as the mixture of gases in the blood each have a pressure. In a mixture of gases, each gas exerts a partial pressure, indicated as PaO_2 for oxygen and $PaCO_2$ for carbon dioxide. The pH of blood is also measured in arterial blood gas analysis.

Arterial blood gas normal values are summarised in the following table.

NAME	NORMAL VALUE
PaO_2	75–100 mmHg
$PaCO_2$	34–45 mmHg
pH	7.35–7.45

Self-assessment test 3.4: summary test

The recap questions below will help to consolidate your learning about the contents of this chapter. Answers can be found at the end of the book.

1   How many milligrams are in 1.3 g?

2   How many milligrams are in 0.8 g?

3   How many milligrams are in 1.125 g?

4   How many milligrams are in 0.6 g?

5   How many milligrams are in 0.505 g?

6   How many micrograms are in 0.75 mg?

7   How many micrograms are in 1.001 mg?

8   How many micrograms are in 0.07 mg?

9   How many micrograms are in 0.902 mg?

Self-assessment test 3.4: summary test (*continued*)

10 How many millilitres are in 1.5 L?

11 How many millilitres are in 2.25 L?

12 How many millilitres are in 0.1 L?

13 How many millilitres are in 0.075 L?

14 How many millilitres are in 0.005 L?

15 What volume of fluid is in the syringe shown?

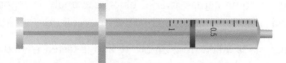

16 What volume of fluid is in the medicine pot shown?

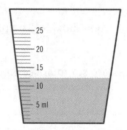

17 Complete the table by converting the SI units.

GRAMS (g)	MILLIGRAMS (mg)	MICROGRAMS
	6	
		120
0.01		
	9.5	
1		
		250
	1	
	2.75	
0.008		
		500

Write your answers to questions 18 to 22 in milligrams.

18 22.5 mg + 4600 micrograms =

19 1.6 mg + 500 micrograms =

20 4.005 mg + 6 micrograms =

21 123 mg – 900 micrograms =

22 6 mg – 25 micrograms =

Self-assessment test 3.4: summary test (*continued*)

23 Place the following weights into ascending order, starting with the smallest. 200 mg, 1100 micrograms, 1.5 g, 5 mg, 65 micrograms, 0.5 g, 0.25 mg, 25 micrograms, 1.5 mg, 0.005 mg, 3 micrograms, 2 g, 2100 mg, 1.6 mg, 1607 micrograms, 750 mg, 0.22 g, 0.034 mg, 0.065 g, 0.125 g, 400 micrograms

24 A patient is prescribed 300 mg of a drug to be taken at breakfast and lunchtime and a dose of 450 mg in the evening. How many grams per day does the patient take?

25 A liquid medicine contains 20 mg in 5 ml.

   a   How many milligrams are in 7.5 ml?

   b   How many milligrams are in 12.5 ml?

26 A patient takes lorazepam 1 mg as sedation before a minor surgical procedure. How many micrograms is this?

27 A patient takes tamsulosin hydrochloride 400 micrograms for benign prostatic hypertrophy. Express this quantity in milligrams.

28 A patient is given 1.5 g of the antibiotic cefuroxime. How many milligrams is this?

29 A patient takes a sodium valproate 300 mg modified release capsule. Express this amount in grams.

30 A patient wears a glyceryl trinitrate 5 mg patch for 24 hours. How many micrograms is this?

KEY POINTS TO TAKE AWAY FROM THIS CHAPTER

- The SI system means that volumes and weights can be written in whole numbers which increases patient safety.
- The strict conventions in the use of abbreviations, plurals and capital letters within the SI system are to ensure accuracy and safety.
- Some units, like mmHg, which is used to measure pressure in clinical practice, are not from the SI system but are acceptable and safe.

04

CALCULATING DRUG DOSES

THIS CHAPTER:

- outlines the rules for administering medicines and the principles used when calculating drug dosages

- explains the methods and equations used when calculating tablet, oral liquid, injection and infusion doses.

4.1 Reducing the risk of administration error

A registered nurse will spend up to a third of each working day on some aspect of administering medicines. The safe administration of medicines is a key nursing role with drug calculations classed as an essential skill. The individual skills that collectively form nursing practice rely on a body of knowledge, or theory. Your knowledge about the theory of performing calculations will have been learnt over many years:

- starting at primary school

- continuing throughout your time at secondary school

- higher levels of study may have further developed your calculation skills.

The mathematics and numeracy qualifications needed to enter a nursing course should help your confidence because you know that under certain conditions you can calculate accurately.

Remember that calculating a drug dose is far more than an arithmetical problem.

It also requires:

- good mentorship to allow you to gain sufficient practical experience

- an awareness of common drug doses

- an understanding of clinical situations that are known to predispose to errors.

PRACTICE TIP

Administering medicines is guided by NHS Trust policy, which incorporates legal and professional requirements.

The procedure involves checking 'the five rights':
- Is it the right medicine?
- Is it the right dose?
- Is it the right time to give the drug?
- Is it via the right route?
- Is it the right patient that I am giving the drug to?

(More details are given in *Appendix 1*.)

RULE OF THUMB

There are basic rules for calculating drug doses:
- The prescribed dose and the available drug must be in the same unit of measurement, so convert if necessary.
- Use an equation and write down each step of the calculation.
- If you are performing a calculation that needs to be checked by another person, make sure you don't show them your answer or working out before they have arrived at an answer independently.
- If a calculation seems extremely complex, discuss this with the prescriber and a pharmacist; there may be a simpler way of arriving at the required dose.

4.2 Calculating for oral administration

Tablets and capsules

Most drug calculations are quite straightforward and can be performed using a 'mental maths' approach and without an obvious need to use a written equation. However, using an equation means that you can demonstrate to another nurse exactly how you arrived at your answer.

The prescription below shows that the patient is prescribed ampicillin 500 mg orally, four times each day.

NAME OF PATIENT:		Elinor Graham				DOB:		13/06/32		
ROUTE	oral	MEDICATION:		Ampicillin		ALLERGIES:		None		
DATE	30/03					DR'S SIGNATURE:		Dr E Wright		
	DOSE	30/03	31/03	01/04	02/04	03/04	04/04	05/04	06/04	
MORNING	500 mg	AD								
MIDDAY	500 mg	AD								
EVENING	500 mg	AD								
BEDTIME	500 mg									

The bedtime dose of 500 mg on 30/03 is due:

- The available capsules are 250 mg

- Use the equation Want (W) ÷ Got (G) = Number of tablets / capsules to be given

  - What you want (W) is the dose

  - What you've got (G) is the amount in each capsule

  - What you need to know is the number of capsules, therefore:

- The dose you want (W) = 500 mg, the amount you have got (G) = 250 mg

- 500 mg ÷ 250 mg = 2 capsules.

Multiplication can also be used in the calculation, particularly to check your answer:

- one capsule equals 250 mg

- two capsules equal 500 mg (i.e., 2 × 250 = 500)

- three capsules equal 750 mg (i.e., 3 × 250 = 750)

- four capsules equal 1000 mg (1 g) (i.e., 4 × 250 = 1000)

and so on.

The prescription below shows that the patient is prescribed warfarin 9 mg orally, each evening.

NAME OF PATIENT:		Don Makepeace			DOB:			01/06/54	
ROUTE	oral	MEDICATION:		Warfarin	ALLERGIES:			None	
DATE	30/03				DR'S SIGNATURE:			Dr E Wright	
	DOSE	30/03	31/03	01/04	02/04	03/04	04/04	05/04	06/04
MORNING									
MIDDAY									
EVENING	9 mg	AD							
BEDTIME									

The evening dose of 9 mg on the 31/03 is due:

- The available tablets are 3 mg (blue tablets)

- Use the equation Want (W) ÷ Got (G) = Number of tablets to be given

    - What you want (W) is the dose

    - What you've got (G) is the amount in each tablet

    - What you need to know is the number of tablets, therefore:

- The dose Wanted = 9 mg, the amount you have Got = 3 mg

- 9 mg ÷ 3 mg = 3 tablets.

Multiplication can also be used in the calculation, particularly to check your answer:

- one tablet equals 3 mg

- two tablets equal 6 mg (i.e., 2 × 3 = 6)

- three tablets equal 9 mg (i.e., 3 × 3 = 9)

- four tablets equal 12 mg (i.e., 4 × 3 = 12)

and so on.

PRACTICE TIP

If your calculation indicates the need to give half a tablet, only tablets that are scored should be cut; ideally the correct strength tablet should be given. Capsules are not suitable for splitting and very small tablets cannot be split in half accurately. Any tablets with a specialised coating such as enteric coating, which is designed to delay the breakdown of the drug, must not be split. Cutting an enteric coated tablet could cause serious harm to a patient.

ERROR ALERT

Some drugs are used to treat different disease processes or clinical features, but at different dosages. An example of this is methotrexate, which can be used as a cytotoxic agent for the treatment of some cancers and can also be used as an immunosuppressant to treat patients with rheumatoid arthritis or psoriasis. It is vital that the patient receives the correct dose, as methotrexate will cause bone marrow depression in toxic doses, which can result in infections and bleeding. So apart from calculating accurately, you need to know (or find out) commonly used dosages and frequency of administration.

When used in the treatment of:
- rheumatoid arthritis or psoriasis, methotrexate is given in amounts less than 25 mg per week
- cancers, doses are higher than 25 mg.

Information about the correct doses and other safety issues are available from:
- the British National Formulary (BNF)
- your local hospital pharmacist
- your ward / departmental dedicated pharmacist.

Self-assessment test 4.1: calculating tablets

The questions below will help to consolidate your learning about calculating the number of tablets to administer. The questions will also get you more familiar with reading prescriptions.

If you are unfamiliar with the drug dosage on a prescription, use a current edition of the BNF to check. You can also clarify the prescription with a pharmacist and the prescriber. A pharmacology book will also give an indication of the typical dosages of commonly used drugs.

Answers can be found at the end of the book.

1 A patient is prescribed 5 mg of bendroflumethiazide to be taken in the morning. How many 2.5 mg tablets should be given?

2 A patient is prescribed 7.5 mg of gastro resistant prednisolone in the morning. How many 2.5 mg tablets should be given?

3 The prescription shows that the patient is prescribed 20 mg of furosemide to be taken at midday on 22/05. How many 40 mg tablets should be given?

NAME OF PATIENT:			Ieuan Graham	DOB:		07/11/67			
ROUTE	oral	MEDICATION:	Furosemide	ALLERGIES:		None			
DATE	22/05			DR'S SIGNATURE:		Dr E Wright			
	DOSE	22/05	23/05	24/05	25/05	26/05	27/05	28/05	29/05
MORNING	40 mg	KW							
MIDDAY	20 mg								
EVENING									
BEDTIME									

4 The prescription shows that the patient is prescribed 250 micrograms of digoxin on the morning of 09/05. How many 125 microgram tablets should be given?

NAME OF PATIENT:			Annette Makepeace	DOB:		21/09/58			
ROUTE	oral	MEDICATION:	Digoxin	ALLERGIES:		None			
DATE	07/05			DR'S SIGNATURE:		Dr E Wright			
	DOSE	07/05	08/05	09/05	10/05	11/05	12/05	13/05	14/05
MORNING	250 micrograms	JD	JD						
MIDDAY									
EVENING									
BEDTIME									

Self-assessment test 4.1: calculating tablets (*continued*)

5 From this prescription, identify the drug, dosage, and time of administration for February 8ᵗʰ.

NAME OF PATIENT:			Bethan Jones		DOB:		18/05/57		
ROUTE	oral	MEDICATION:	Gliclazide		ALLERGIES:		None		
DATE	07/02				DR'S SIGNATURE:		Dr E Wright		
	DOSE	07/02	08/02	09/02	10/02	11/02	12/02	13/02	14/02
MORNING	40 mg	AD							
MIDDAY									
EVENING									
BEDTIME									

6 From this prescription, identify the drug, dosage and time that the drug is next due to be given.

NAME OF PATIENT:			Kate Wilson		DOB:		07/02/51		
ROUTE	oral	MEDICATION:	Metoprolol		ALLERGIES:		None		
DATE	12/02				DR'S SIGNATURE:		Dr E Wright		
	DOSE	12/02	13/02	14/02	15/02	16/02	17/02	18/02	19/02
MORNING	50 mg	HD	HD	HD	KW				
MIDDAY	50 mg	JP	JP	SD	JP				
EVENING									
BEDTIME	50 mg	KW	WP	KW					

7 A prescription shows that the patient, a 75-year-old female, is due for her levothyroxine sodium. This is given once daily as she has an under-functioning thyroid, diagnosed 7 years ago. 100 mg of levothyroxine sodium is prescribed to be given in the morning, but the stock tablets are 25 micrograms and you suspect that this dose is too high. A quick calculation tells you that you would need 4000 of the 25 microgram tablets for a 100 mg dose. Do you think that 100 mg is the correct dose? If not, what is the typical dose range for this patient?

Self-assessment test 4.1: calculating tablets (*continued*)

8 Read the following prescription carefully; it shows that the patient is prescribed 7.5 mg of zopiclone used for short-term insomnia, to be given on 13/06. Do you need to check the prescription with the prescriber? If so, why?

NAME OF PATIENT:				David Mathews		DOB:		12/07/24	
ROUTE	oral	MEDICATION:		Zopiclone		ALLERGIES:		None	
DATE	13/06					DR'S SIGNATURE:		Dr E Wright	
	DOSE	13/06	14/06	15/06	16/06	17/06	18/06	19/06	20/06
MORNING	7.5 mg								
MIDDAY									
EVENING									
BEDTIME									

ERROR ALERT

Not all calculation errors are caused by mathematical mistakes. Some drugs are calculated by automated dosage software like the INRstar system.

The INRstar system:

- is widely used in GP surgeries for anticoagulant management
- calculates patients' INR (International Normalised Ratio) which is a measurement of the time taken for blood to form a clot
- calculates anticoagulant dosages.

The INRstar software assumes that patients take all of their prescribed anticoagulant such as warfarin, and that no doses are missed. If a patient misses a dose and doesn't report this, then the software may advise a higher dose to maintain the correct INR. This is because the software 'thinks' that if the patient is taking the prescribed dose and the INR has fallen slightly, then a higher dose will keep it at the correct level. However, the reality is that the patient has taken a lower dose than the one prescribed. The result is an unnecessary increase in warfarin leading to a potentially dangerous rise in their INR level.

Liquid medicines

Two different processes can be used to calculate the amount of a liquid medicine to administer. One method uses a ratio approach and one uses an equation.

The ratio approach

This method involves finding out how many milligrams each millilitre contains.

For example:

- A patient is prescribed morphine solution (Oramorph) 8 mg.

- The solution contains 10 mg in 5 ml.

- What you want to know is how many mg there are in 1 ml.

- To find this out, divide the 10 (mg) by 5 (ml).

- 10 ÷ 5 = 2, so each ml of solution contains 2 mg of morphine.

- The required dose is 8 mg and the solution we have contains 2 mg per ml.

Using a ratio approach we can explain that if there are 2 mg in 1 ml, there are 4 mg in 2 ml, 6 mg in 3 ml and 8 mg in 4 ml. The following table shows this visually:

mg	ml
2	1
4	2
6	3
8	4

So for a dose of 8 mg, it is necessary to administer 4 ml of morphine solution because 4 (ml) × 2 (mg) = 8 mg.

SENSE CHECK

The patient is prescribed 8 mg and 5 ml of solution contains 10 mg – so you know that you need less than 5 ml to administer 8 mg.

The equation

There are several versions of the equation that can be used, but one of the most commonly applied ones is known as the 'WIG' equation.

'WIG' stands for 'Want, In, Got'.

- What you 'Want' is the amount of drug prescribed.

- What it is 'In' is the volume that the drug is contained in.

- What you have 'Got' is the strength of the solution.

The WIG equation is written as:

$$\frac{\text{What you } \textbf{WANT} \times \text{What it is } \textbf{IN}}{\text{What you have } \textbf{GOT}}$$

This equation instructs you to multiply the required drug dose (Want) by the amount it is in (In), and then divide this by the strength of the drug available (Got).

EXAMPLE 4.1

Using the previous Oramorph example:
- The patient is prescribed morphine solution (Oramorph) 8 mg.
- The solution contains 10 mg in 5 ml.
- Using the WIG equation:
  - What you want is 8 mg
  - What it's in is 5 ml
  - What you've got is 10 mg.

The prescribed dose and the available drug are in the same units (mg), so no conversion is necessary. The equation can be written as:

$$\frac{(\text{What you want) } 8 \times (\text{What it's in) } 5}{(\text{What you've got) } 10} = \frac{40}{10} = 4 \, \text{ml}$$

EXAMPLE 4.2

A patient is prescribed diazepam elixir 10 mg. The label indicates that the stock available contains 5 mg in 5 ml.
- Using the WIG equation:
  - What you want is 10 mg
  - What it's in is 5 ml
  - What you've got is 5 mg.

So the equation can be written as:

$$\frac{(\text{What you want) } 10 \times (\text{What it's in) } 5}{(\text{What you've got) } 5} = \frac{50}{5} = 10 \, \text{ml of diazepam elixir should be given}$$

Checking the calculation with the ratio approach

A patient is prescribed diazepam elixir 10 mg.
- The solution contains 5 mg in 5 ml.
- What you want to know is how many mg there are in 1 ml.
- To find this out, divide the 5 (mg) by 5 (ml).
- 5 ÷ 5 = 1, so each ml of solution contains 1 mg of diazepam.
- The required dose is 10 mg and the solution we have contains 1 mg per ml.

Using a ratio approach we can explain that if there is 1 mg in 1 ml, there are 5 mg in 5 ml and 10 mg in 10 ml. The following table shows this visually:

mg	ml
1	1
5	5
10	10

EXAMPLE 4.3

A patient is prescribed sodium valproate liquid 400 mg. The label indicates that the stock available contains 200 mg in 5 ml.
- Using the WIG equation:
  - What you want is 400 mg
  - What it's in is 5 ml
  - What you've got is 200 mg.

So the equation can be written as:

$$\frac{(\text{What you want}) \, 400 \times (\text{What it's in}) \, 5}{(\text{What you've got}) \, 200} = \frac{2000}{200} = \begin{array}{l} 10 \, \text{ml of sodium valproate} \\ \text{liquid should be given} \end{array}$$

Checking the calculation with the ratio approach

A patient is prescribed sodium valproate liquid 400 mg.
- The solution contains 200 mg in 5 ml.
- What you want to know is how many mg there are in 1 ml.
- To find this out, divide the 200 (mg) by 5 (ml).
- 200 ÷ 5 = 40, so each ml of solution contains 40 mg of sodium valproate.
- The required dose is 400 mg and the solution we have contains 40 mg per ml.

Using a ratio approach we can explain that if there are 40 mg in 1 ml, there are 400 mg in 10 ml. The following table shows this visually:

mg	ml
40	1
80	2
120	3
160	4
200	5
240	6
280	7
320	8
360	9
400	10

EXAMPLE 4.4

A patient is prescribed 1 g of metformin syrup. The label indicates that the stock available contains 500 mg in 5 ml.
- Using the WIG equation:
  - What you want is 1 g
  - What it's in is 5 ml
  - What you've got is 500 mg.

In this example the amount of drug prescribed and the available drug are in different units of measurement. One of the rules of thumb for calculating dosages states that 'the prescribed dose and the available drug must be in the same unit of measurement, so convert if necessary'. In this case we have metformin 1 g prescribed and 500 mg in 5 ml available so we need to convert into the smaller of the two units of measurement – mg.

- Using the WIG equation:
  - What you want is 1000 mg (because 1 g = 1000 mg)
  - What it's in is 5 ml
  - What you've got is 500 mg.

So the equation can be written as:

$$\frac{(\text{What you want}) \ 1000 \times (\text{What it's in}) \ 5}{(\text{What you've got}) \ 500} = \frac{5000}{500} = \frac{10 \ \text{ml of metformin syrup}}{\text{should be given}}$$

Checking the calculation with the ratio approach

A patient is prescribed metformin syrup 1 g.
- The solution contains 500 mg in 5 ml.
- What you want to know is how many mg there are in 1 ml.
- To find this out, divide the 500 (mg) by 5 (ml).
- 500 ÷ 5 = 100, so each ml of solution contains 100 mg of metformin.
- The required dose is 1 g or 1000 mg and the solution we have contains 100 mg per ml.

Using a ratio approach we can explain that if there is 100 mg in 1 ml, there are 500 mg in 5 ml and 1000 mg or 1 g in 10 ml. The following table shows this visually:

mg	ml
100	1
500	5
1000	10

ERROR ALERT

Examining past drug errors has identified that oral medicines and nebuliser solutions have sometimes been inadvertently administered intravenously. To avoid similar errors, don't take drugs that need to be given by different routes to a patient at the same time and double check the route of administration during the procedure. Remember that the route is one of the five 'rights'.

Self-assessment test 4.2: calculating liquid medicines

The questions below will help to consolidate your learning about calculating volumes of liquid medicines. Answers can be found at the end of the book.

1 A patient is prescribed 10 mg of amiloride oral solution. The oral solution contains 5 mg in 5 ml, how many millilitres should be given?

2 A patient is prescribed 500 mg of ampicillin oral suspension. The oral suspension contains 250 mg in 5 ml, how many millilitres should be given?

3 The prescription shows that the patient is prescribed 150 mg of amantadine to be given in the evening on 22/05. The oral solution contains 50 mg in 5 ml, how many millilitres should be given?

NAME OF PATIENT:			Maurice Booker		DOB:		11/07/63		
ROUTE	oral	MEDICATION:	Amantadine		ALLERGIES:		None		
DATE	22/05		syrup		DR'S SIGNATURE:		Dr E Wright		
	DOSE	22/05	23/05	24/05	25/05	26/05	27/05	28/05	29/05
MORNING	150 mg	KW							
MIDDAY									
EVENING	150 mg								
BEDTIME									

4 The prescription shows that the patient is prescribed 80 mg of furosemide to be given in the morning on 08/05. The oral solution contains 20 mg in 5 ml, how many millilitres should be given?

NAME OF PATIENT:			Florence Facer		DOB:		09/02/30		
ROUTE	oral	MEDICATION:	Furosemide		ALLERGIES:		None		
DATE	07/05		oral solution		DR'S SIGNATURE:		Dr E Wright		
	DOSE	07/05	08/05	09/05	10/05	11/05	12/05	13/05	14/05
MORNING	80 mg	JD							
MIDDAY									
EVENING									
BEDTIME									

Self-assessment test 4.2: calculating liquid medicines (*continued*)

5 From this prescription, identify the drug, dosage and volume (the oral solution contains 2 mg in 5 ml) and time that the drug is next due on September 22nd.

NAME OF PATIENT:			Donald Walter		DOB:		17/02/82		
ROUTE	oral	MEDICATION:	Diazepam oral solution		ALLERGIES:		None		
DATE	21/09				DR'S SIGNATURE:		Dr E Wright		
	DOSE	21/09	22/09	23/09	24/09	25/09	26/09	27/09	28/09
MORNING	4 mg	AD	AD						
MIDDAY	4 mg	AD							
EVENING									
BEDTIME	4 mg	AD							

6 From this prescription, identify the volume of levothyroxine due to be given on the morning of 31/07. The oral solution contains 50 micrograms in 5 ml.

NAME OF PATIENT:			John Grantham		DOB:		17/08/89		
ROUTE	oral	MEDICATION:	Levothyroxine oral solution		ALLERGIES:		None		
DATE	28/07				DR'S SIGNATURE:		Dr E Wright		
	DOSE	28/07	29/07	30/07	31/07	01/08	02/08	03/08	04/08
MORNING	150 micrograms	HD	HD	HD					
MIDDAY									
EVENING									
BEDTIME									

7 A prescription shows that an adult female patient is prescribed 1400 mg of ferrous fumarate to be given twice daily. The oral solution contains 140 mg in 5 ml, and you calculate that a dose of 50 ml is needed for each dose but are concerned that this seems a large amount. You haven't given iron as an oral solution before but can recall giving 200 mg iron tablets to a patient. What is the appropriate dose for the patient?

Self-assessment test 4.2: calculating liquid medicines (*continued*)

8 The prescription shows that a patient diagnosed with high blood pressure has been prescribed propranolol. The drug is to be started on the morning of 22/05. 10 mg of propranolol are prescribed and the oral solution contains 10 mg in 5 ml. You notice that the stock tablets used for a different patient contain 40 mg each. Do you need to check this prescription with the prescriber? If so, why?

NAME OF PATIENT:			Vicki Fenn		DOB:		13/08/56			
ROUTE	oral	MEDICATION:	Propranolol		ALLERGIES:		None			
DATE	22/05		oral solution		DR'S SIGNATURE:		Dr E Wright			
	DOSE	22/05	23/05	24/05	25/05	26/05	27/05	28/05	29/05
MORNING	10 mg								
MIDDAY									
EVENING	10 mg								
BEDTIME									

4.3 Calculating for administration by injection

The WIG equation is an essential tool for calculating the volume of a drug to be injected.

EXAMPLE 4.5

A patient is prescribed hydrocortisone 40 mg as an intramuscular injection. Ampoules containing 50 mg in 2 ml are available. Calculate the volume required for the injection.

- Use the WIG equation:

- The patient is prescribed hydrocortisone 40 mg.
- The ampoules contain 50 mg in 2 ml.
- Using the WIG equation:
  - What you want is 40 mg
  - What it's in is 2 ml
  - What you've got is 50 mg.

So the equation can be written as:

$$\frac{\text{(What you want) } 40 \times \text{(What it's in) } 2}{\text{(What you've got) } 50} = \frac{80}{50} = 1.6 \, \text{ml}$$

EXAMPLE 4.6

A patient is prescribed furosemide 35 mg as an intramuscular injection. Ampoules containing 50 mg in 5 ml are available. Calculate the volume required for the injection.

- Use the WIG equation: $\dfrac{\text{What you WANT} \times \text{What it is IN}}{\text{What you have GOT}}$
- The patient is prescribed furosemide 35 mg.
- The ampoules contain 50 mg in 5 ml.
- Using the WIG equation:
  - What you want is 35 mg
  - What it's in is 5 ml
  - What you've got is 50 mg.

So the equation can be written as:

$$\frac{\text{(What you want) } 35 \times \text{(What it's in) } 5}{\text{(What you've got) } 50} = \frac{175}{50} = 3.5 \, \text{ml}$$

Self-assessment test 4.3: calculating injections

The recap questions below will help to consolidate your understanding about calculating injections using the WIG equation. Answers can be found at the end of the book.

1 A patient is prescribed teicoplanin 400 mg as an intramuscular injection. When the vial is reconstituted there are 200 mg per ml. What volume needs to be injected?

2 A patient is prescribed gentamicin 100 mg as an intramuscular injection. Ampoules contain 40 mg / ml. Calculate the volume to be injected.

3 The prescription shows that the patient is due to receive 15 mg of morphine by intramuscular injection in the evening on 22/03. Ampoules contain 10 mg / ml. Calculate the volume to be injected.

NAME OF PATIENT:			William Kelsey		DOB:		06/11/82			
ROUTE	IM injection	MEDICATION:		Morphine	ALLERGIES:		None			
DATE	22/03				DR'S SIGNATURE:		Dr E Wright			
	DOSE	22/03	23/03	24/03	25/03	26/03	27/03	28/03	29/03
MORNING	15 mg	KW							
MIDDAY	15 mg	NAD							
EVENING	15 mg								
BEDTIME	15 mg								

Self-assessment test 4.3: calculating injections (*continued*)

4 A patient is prescribed ampicillin 500 mg as an intramuscular injection due to be given at midday on 03/11. When the vial is reconstituted there are 250 mg per ml. What volume needs to be injected?

NAME OF PATIENT:			Hilda Wright		DOB:		12/09/32		
ROUTE	IM injection	MEDICATION:	Ampicillin		ALLERGIES:		None		
DATE	02/11				DR'S SIGNATURE:		Dr E Wright		
	DOSE	02/11	03/11	04/11	05/11	06/11	07/11	08/11	09/11
MORNING	500 mg	KW	NAD						
MIDDAY	500 mg	NAD							
EVENING	500 mg	AD							
BEDTIME	500 mg	NT							

5 From this prescription, identify the drug, dosage and volume to be given at bedtime on 22/09. Ampoules contain 10 mg / ml.

NAME OF PATIENT:			Anne Williams		DOB:		22/05/60		
ROUTE	IM injection	MEDICATION:	Furosemide		ALLERGIES:		None		
DATE	21/09				DR'S SIGNATURE:		Dr E Wright		
	DOSE	21/09	22/09	23/09	24/09	25/09	26/09	27/09	28/09
MORNING	25 mg	AD	SD						
MIDDAY	25 mg	NAD	KG						
EVENING									
BEDTIME	25 mg	AD							

6 From this prescription, identify the drug, dosage and volume to be given in the evening on 22/05. Ampoules contain 50 mg / ml.

NAME OF PATIENT:			Angharad Williams		DOB:		12/02/85		
ROUTE	IM injection	MEDICATION:	Dihydrocodeine		ALLERGIES:		None		
DATE	21/05				DR'S SIGNATURE:		Dr E Wright		
	DOSE	21/05	22/05	23/05	24/05	25/05	26/05	27/05	28/05
MORNING	40 mg	AD	EC						
MIDDAY	40 mg	FN	MS						
EVENING	40 mg	FN							
BEDTIME	40 mg	BC							

7 A prescription shows that an adult male patient diagnosed with bradycardia is prescribed 3 mg of atropine by intramuscular injection. Ampoules contain 600 micrograms / ml. How many ampoules would be necessary for a 3 mg dose? What is the appropriate dose for the patient?

Self-assessment test 4.3: calculating injections (*continued*)

8 Read the following prescription carefully; it shows that the patient is prescribed 2 g of hydrocortisone, to be given in the morning of 13/06. Do you need to check the prescription with the prescriber? If so, why?

NAME OF PATIENT:			Jack Davison			DOB:		07/05/88	
ROUTE	IM injection	MEDICATION:	Hydro-cortisone			ALLERGIES:		None	
DATE	13/06					DR'S SIGNATURE:		Dr E Wright	
	DOSE	13/06	14/06	15/06	16/06	17/06	18/06	19/06	20/06
MORNING	2 g								
MIDDAY	2 g								
EVENING	2 g								
BEDTIME	2 g								

4.4 Calculating intravenous infusions

Intravenous flow rates

The flow rate is the speed at which a volume of fluid is given intravenously to a patient over a given period of time. Flow rates are an important clinical calculation and crucial in ensuring patient safety. The administration of intravenous fluids and additives is a very common intervention across many clinical environments. Infusing fluids too rapidly can harm elderly patients or those with heart disease, whereas too little fluid may result in dehydration.

> **ERROR ALERT**
>
> Many intravenous fluids contain numbers as part of their name, for example glucose 5% and sodium chloride 0.9%. The numbers indicate the concentration of substances in the intravenous fluid and do not play a role within any drug or flow rate calculation.

Flow rates are calculated by dividing the volume of intravenous fluid to be infused, by the number of hours that the infusion is prescribed to run over. The result gives the number of millilitres to be infused per hour.

$$\frac{\text{Volume to be infused (ml)}}{\text{Duration of infusion (hours)}} = \text{ml per hour}$$

EXAMPLE 4.7

A patient is to receive 1000 ml of Ringer's solution over 5 hours.
- 1000 ÷ 5 = 200 ml / hour

EXAMPLE 4.8

A patient is to receive 500 ml of sodium chloride 0.9% over 8 hours.
- 500 ÷ 8 = 62.5 ml / hour

Sometimes these calculations will result in a recurring decimal number.

EXAMPLE 4.9

A patient is to be given 500 ml of glucose 5% over 3 hours.
- 500 ÷ 3 = 166.6666666666 ml / hour
- The '.666666666' part of the number is recurring and to save writing out long numbers like this, there is an abbreviation system.
- 166.666666666 can be abbreviated to:
  - 166.6 r or 166.666... or 166.6̇

EXAMPLE 4.10

A patient is to receive 500 ml of dextrose 4% saline 0.18% over 6 hours.
- 500 ÷ 6 = 83.3333333333 ml / hour
- The '.3333333333' part of the number is recurring and can be abbreviated to:
  - 83.3r or 83.333... or 83.3̇

PRACTICE TIP

An electronic volumetric pump can be used to control intravenous infusions of patients who may be at risk from over or under infusion, or who are receiving additives or drugs via the infusion. Manually calculating the flow rate of an intravenous infusion is an essential step when checking the safe functioning of a volumetric pump.

ERROR ALERT

Intravenous drug calculations follow the same rules as other injections. As there are two calculations to be performed, the dose of the drug and the rate of infusion, there are two potential sources of error.

Self-assessment test 4.4: calculating intravenous flow rates

The recap questions below will help to consolidate your understanding of calculating intravenous flow rates. Answers can be found at the end of the book.

1 A patient is to receive 500 ml of sodium chloride 0.9% over 4 hours. How many ml per hour will be infused?

2 A patient is to receive 500 ml of dextrose 5% over 2 hours. How many ml per hour will be infused?

3 A patient is to receive 1000 ml of Ringer's solution over 8 hours. How many ml per hour will be infused?

4 A patient is to receive 500 ml of dextrose 5% over 8 hours. How many ml are still to be infused after 3 hours?

5 A patient is to receive 500 ml of sodium chloride 0.9% over 10 hours. How many ml are still to be infused after 7 hours?

6 A patient is to receive 1000 ml of sodium chloride 0.9% over 8 hours. How many ml are still to be infused after 5 hours?

7 A patient is to receive 500 ml of Ringer's solution over 5 hours. How many ml are still to be infused after 3 hours?

8 A patient is to receive 1000 ml of sodium chloride 0.9% over 8 hours. After 6 hours, how many ml have been infused?

9 A patient is to receive 500 ml of dextrose 5% over 4 hours. After 1 hour, how many ml have been infused?

10 A patient is to receive 1000 ml of sodium chloride 0.9% over 4 hours. After 2.5 hours, how many ml have been infused?

Intravenous infusion drop rates

All patients receiving intravenous fluids need careful observation. Simple fluids without additives or drugs can be administered through a standard intravenous giving set. This doesn't need an electronic pump or device to control the flow of the intravenous fluid as this is done by adjusting the number of drops of fluid per minute (drops per minute) in the intravenous giving set. The more drops per minute observed in the chamber of the giving set, the higher the flow rate of intravenous fluid into the patient.

It is necessary to be able to calculate the number of drops per minute as this tells us how many ml per hour are being infused.

A standard intravenous administration set has 20 drops per ml (blood administration sets have 15 drops per ml).

To calculate the flow rate of an intravenous infusion, we need to know:

• the volume of fluid to be infused in ml

• the length of time for the infusion

• the drops per ml of the intravenous giving set.

The equation to calculate the number of drops per minute is:

$$\frac{\text{Volume prescribed (ml)}}{\text{Hours of infusion}} \times \frac{\text{Drops per ml of administration set}}{\text{60 minutes}}$$

To calculate the volume of fluid required every hour, you divide the volume by hours.

To calculate the number of drops needed to administer that volume in one hour, you multiply by the number of drops per ml.

To calculate the number of drops needed per minute, divide by 60 (there are 60 minutes in one hour).

EXAMPLE 4.11

A patient is prescribed 500 ml of sodium chloride 0.9% intravenously over 4 hours.
• The volume of fluid to be infused = 500
• The length of time for the infusion = 4
• The drops per ml of the intravenous giving set = 20

Inserting these figures into the equation gives:

$$\frac{500}{4} \times \frac{20}{60} = 125 \times 0.33\,r = 41.66\,r$$

Note: We can't give 41.66 r drops per minute, as we're unable to measure 0.66 r of a drop. So we have to infuse either 42 or 41 drops per minute. If we infused 42 drops per minute, this might lead to over infusion and the intravenous giving set might empty of fluid, leading to air entering the set and tubing. Therefore we round down to the nearest whole number and administer 41 drops per minute.

EXAMPLE 4.12

A patient is prescribed 1000 ml of Ringer's solution intravenously over 12 hours.
• The volume of fluid to be infused = 1000
• The length of time for the infusion = 12
• The drops per ml of the intravenous giving set = 20

Inserting these figures into the equation gives:

$$\frac{1000}{12} \times \frac{20}{60} = 83.3r \times 0.33r = 27.77r = 27 \text{ drops per minute}$$

> **PRACTICE TIP**
>
> In maths there is a general principle about 'rounding off' numbers where a high degree of precision isn't required. Numbers including five or more round up, and four or less round down.
> - The number 9.57 correct to one decimal place is rounded up to 9.6
> - The digit '7' in the second decimal place is equal to or greater than five, so rounds up making the digit '5' in the first decimal place into a '6'.
> - Similarly, 9.54 correct to one decimal place becomes 9.5 because the digit '4' in the second decimal place is equal to four or less and therefore rounds down, resulting in 9.5.

When performing drops per minute (or ml per hour) calculations for intravenous infusions, don't use the mathematical rounding off principle. In *Example 4.11* where a patient needed to receive 41.66r drops per minute, mathematically this would be rounded up to 42 drops per minute. In clinical practice this could result in the infusion running slightly too fast and air entering the administration set, both threatening patient safety.

Blood transfusion drop rates

Intravenous giving sets used for blood transfusions are different to those used for other fluids and contain 15 drops per ml.

To calculate the flow rate of a blood transfusion, the same information is needed:

- the volume to be infused in ml

- the length of time for the infusion

- the drops per ml of the intravenous giving set.

The equation to calculate the number of drops per minute is the same as for intravenous fluids:

$$\frac{\text{Volume prescribed (ml)}}{\text{Hours of infusion}} \times \frac{\text{Drops per ml of administration set}}{\text{60 minutes}}$$

EXAMPLE 4.13

A patient is prescribed a transfusion of whole blood (500 ml) over 2 hours.
- The volume of fluid to be infused = 500
- The length of time for the infusion = 2
- The drops per ml of the intravenous giving set = 15

Inserting these figures into the equation gives:

$$\frac{500}{2} \times \frac{15}{60} = 250 \times 0.25 = 62.5 \text{ drops per minute}$$

EXAMPLE 4.14

A patient is prescribed a transfusion of whole blood (500 ml) over 1 hour.
- The volume of fluid to be infused = 500
- The length of time for the infusion = 1
- The drops per ml of the intravenous giving set = 15

Inserting these figures into the equation gives:

$$\frac{500}{1} \times \frac{15}{60} = 500 \times 0.25 = 125 \text{ drops per minute}$$

PRACTICE TIP

Be aware that blood isn't always given in standardised bags of 500 ml. Sometimes the volume is less than this if the patient needs the cellular part of the blood more than the fluid.

Self-assessment test 4.5: calculating intravenous infusion drop rates

The recap questions below will help to consolidate your skill of calculating intravenous infusion drop rates. Some of the later questions are more challenging; a description of the processes followed can be found as part of the answers at the end of the book.

1 A patient is prescribed 1000 ml of intravenous Ringer's solution to run over 6 hours. Using a standard intravenous infusion set, how many drops per minute are needed to infuse the fluid over the prescribed time?

2 A patient is prescribed 500 ml of intravenous sodium chloride 0.9% to run over 3 hours. Using a standard intravenous infusion set, how many drops per minute are needed to infuse the fluid over the prescribed time?

Self-assessment test 4.5: calculating intravenous infusion drop rates (*continued*)

3   A patient is prescribed 500 ml of intravenous Ringer's solution to run over 5 hours. Using a standard intravenous infusion set, how many drops per minute are needed to infuse the fluid over the prescribed time?

4   A patient is prescribed 500 ml of intravenous glucose 5% to run over 2 hours. Using a standard intravenous infusion set, how many drops per minute are needed to infuse the fluid over the prescribed time?

5   A patient is prescribed 500 ml of intravenous sodium chloride 0.9% to run over 4 hours. Using a standard intravenous infusion set, how many drops per minute are needed to infuse the fluid over the prescribed time?

6   A patient is prescribed 1000 ml of intravenous sodium chloride 0.9% to run over 8 hours. Using a standard intravenous infusion set, how many drops per minute are needed to infuse the fluid over the prescribed time?

7   A patient is prescribed 1000 ml of intravenous sodium chloride 0.9% to run over 12 hours. Using a standard intravenous infusion set, how many drops per minute are needed to infuse the fluid over the prescribed time?

8   A patient is prescribed 500 ml of intravenous glucose 5% to run over 6 hours, using a standard intravenous infusion set. After 3 hours the patient's condition changes and the remaining fluid needs to be infused over 2 hours. How many drops per minute are needed to infuse the remaining fluid over the newly prescribed time?

9   A patient is prescribed 1000 ml of intravenous glucose 5% to run over 9 hours. After 4.5 hours the patient's condition changes and the remaining fluid needs to be infused over 3 hours. How many drops per minute are needed to infuse the remaining fluid over the newly prescribed time?

10 A patient is prescribed 500 ml of intravenous sodium chloride 0.9% to run over 10 hours. After 1 hour the patient's condition changes and the remaining fluid needs to be infused over 5 hours. How many drops per minute are needed to infuse the remaining fluid over the newly prescribed time?

11 A patient is prescribed a transfusion of 500 ml of whole blood to run over 3 hours. How many drops per minute are needed to ensure that the transfusion runs to time?

12 A patient is prescribed a transfusion of 500 ml of whole blood to run over 4 hours. How many drops per minute are needed to ensure that the transfusion runs to time?

> **PRACTICE TIP**
>
> It's important to know the formula and be able to calculate the number of drops per minute correctly. Once you know the number of drops per ml for the administration sets that you are using in your area of clinical practice, there is a short-cut that you can use.
>
> For a blood administration set:
> * Instead of dividing 15 drops per ml by 60, replace this with 4
>
> For a standard administration set:
> * Instead of dividing 20 drops per ml by 60 minutes, replace this with 3
>
> The calculation in *Example 4.11* using a standard administration set then becomes:
>
> $$\frac{500}{4} \times \frac{1}{3} = 125 \div 3 = 41.66\,\text{r drops per minute}$$

4.5 Drug calculations based on per kilogram of body weight

Some drugs, particularly in paediatrics, are prescribed per kilogram of the patient's body weight. There are several reasons for this:

* The breakdown and excretion of drugs in children under 6 months is not as effective as in older children, so lower doses will need to be prescribed.

* As a precaution against adult-sized doses being prescribed where this would be harmful.

* Where a drug has a short duration of action and would need to be infused continuously, for example lidocaine – a drug used intravenously for some heart conditions.

The prescription will state the number of micrograms or milligrams per kilogram of body weight, so the calculation is:

* Microgram or mg × patient's body weight in kg

If the drug is prescribed as millilitres per kilogram, the calculation becomes:

* ml × patient's body weight in kg

The equation can be written as:

* Dose to be administered = dose per kg × patient's body weight in kg

EXAMPLE 4.15

A patient is prescribed gentamicin 4 mg / kg of body weight daily, to be given in three equal doses over 24 hours. The patient weighs 81 kg. The stock ampoules of gentamicin contain 80 mg in 2 ml.
So the equation is:

   dose per kg (4) × patient's body weight (81 kg)

or

   4 × 81 = 324 mg

(This is the total daily amount of gentamicin that is given in three divided doses.)

To calculate the individual doses, 324 mg needs to be divided by 3:

   324 ÷ 3 = 108

Therefore each dose is 108 mg.

This provides the number of milligrams required in each dose, but in addition to this it is necessary to calculate the volume that needs drawing up into a syringe. Gentamicin is stocked in vials of 80 mg in 2 ml.

To calculate the amount to be given, use the WIG equation.
- Using the WIG equation:
  - What you want is 108 mg
  - What it's in is 2 ml
  - What you've got is 80 mg.

So the equation can be written as:

$$\frac{\text{(What you want) } 108 \times \text{(What it's in) } 2}{\text{(What you've got) } 80} = \frac{216}{80} = 2.7 \text{ ml}$$

Drug calculations based on per kilogram of body weight per minute / hour

On occasions, a drug is prescribed per kilogram of body weight over a set period of time. This is only possible to achieve by continuous intravenous infusion via a volumetric pump:

- the dose will be prescribed as mg or microgram / kg / hr.

EXAMPLE 4.16

The drug flecainide is used in the treatment of some heart conditions where there are irregularities in the rhythm. It is available in 15 ml ampoules containing 10 mg / ml. A patient weighing 70 kg is prescribed 100 micrograms of flecainide per kg per hour to be given by continuous intravenous infusion for 12 hours.
- 100 (micrograms) × 70 (kg) per hour
- 100 × 70 micrograms per hour = 7000 micrograms / hr

This is the hourly amount of drug being infused, so to calculate the amount needed for the 12-hour period:
- 12 × 7000 micrograms are to be given = 84 000 micrograms

To calculate the volume of flecainide to be drawn up into a syringe and added to the infusion fluid, 84 000 micrograms needs converting into mg as this is the unit that the drug is available in.
As there are 1000 micrograms in each mg:
- 84 000 ÷ 1000 = 84 mg

The ampoules of flecainide contain 10 mg / ml.

The amount to be drawn up into the syringe can be calculated using the WIG equation.
- Using the WIG equation:
  - What you want is 84 mg
  - What it's in is 15 ml
  - What you've got is 150 mg (15 ml of 10 mg / ml).

So the equation can be written as:

$$\frac{(\text{What you want})\ 84 \times (\text{What it's in})\ 15}{(\text{What you've got})\ 150} = \frac{1260}{150} = 8.4\,\text{ml}$$

So 8.4 ml of flecainide needs to be drawn up from the 15 ml contained in the ampoule.

EXAMPLE 4.17

The drug dopamine is used in the treatment of cardiogenic shock, a serious heart condition. It is available in 5 ml ampoules containing 160 mg / ml.
A patient weighing 80 kg is prescribed 5 micrograms of dopamine per kg per minute to be given by continuous intravenous infusion for 10 hours.
- 5 (micrograms) × 80 (kg) per minute
- 5 × 80 micrograms per minute = 400 micrograms / minute

To calculate the hourly amount of dopamine being given, the amount per minute needs to be multiplied by 60:

- 400 × 60 = 24 000 micrograms per hour

This is the hourly amount of drug being infused, so to calculate the amount needed for the 10-hour period:

- 10 × 24 000 micrograms are to be given = 240 000 micrograms

To calculate the volume of dopamine to be drawn up into a syringe and added to the infusion fluid, 240 000 micrograms needs converting into mg as this is the unit that the drug is available in.

As there are 1000 micrograms in each mg:

- 240 000 ÷ 1000 = 240 mg

The 5 ml ampoules of dopamine contain 160 mg / ml.

The amount to be drawn up into the syringe can be calculated using the WIG equation:

What you **WANT** × What it is **IN**
    What you have **GOT**

- Using the WIG equation:
  - What you want is 240 mg
  - What it's in is 5 ml
  - What you've got is 800 mg (5 ml of 160 mg / ml).

So the equation can be written as:

$$\frac{(\text{What you want})\ 240 \times (\text{What it's in})\ 5}{(\text{What you've got})\ 800} = \frac{1200}{800} = 1.5\,\text{ml}$$

So 1.5 ml of dopamine needs to be drawn up from the 5 ml contained in the ampoule.

ERROR ALERT

Calculations for drugs based on body weight involve at least two mathematical procedures. This means there are at least two potential sources of error in this type of calculation.

Self-assessment test 4.6: calculating dose per kilogram of body weight

The recap questions below will help to consolidate your understanding of performing calculations per kilogram of body weight. Answers can be found at the end of the book.

1   A patient weighing 72 kg is prescribed gentamicin 5 mg per kg of body weight daily.

    a   **What is the total daily amount of gentamicin to be given?**

    b   **If there are three equal doses per day, how many milligrams of gentamicin are given at each dose?**

2   A child weighs 37.5 kg and is prescribed diclofenac sodium orally 2 mg per kilogram of body weight daily in three divided doses.

    a   **What is the total amount of diclofenac sodium given over 24 hours?**

    b   **How many milligrams are in each of the three doses?**

3   A patient weighing 86 kg is prescribed atenolol 150 micrograms per kg intravenously over 20 minutes.

    a   **How many micrograms will be given?**

    b   **Convert your answer to mg.**

4   A patient weighing 70 kg is prescribed an injection of midazolam intramuscularly at 80 microgram per kilogram of body weight.

    a   **What amount of midazolam needs to be given?**

    b   **Convert your answer to mg.**

5   A patient weighing 68 kg is prescribed dopamine 5 micrograms per kilogram per minute by continuous intravenous infusion.

    a   **How many micrograms of dopamine need to be given each minute?**

    b   **If the stock dopamine is 40 mg / ml, how many millilitres will be used over a 24-hour period?**

ERROR ALERT

Calculations like these are classed as complex and demand that two nurses read the prescription and perform the calculation to avoid a serious overdose.

Self-assessment test 4.7: summary test

The questions below will help to consolidate your learning about the contents of this chapter. Answers can be found at the end of the book.

1 A patient is prescribed 1g of paracetamol. How many 500 mg tablets should be given?

2 A patient is prescribed 7.5 mg of soluble prednisolone orally. How many 5 mg tablets should be given?

3 A patient is prescribed 250 micrograms of digoxin. How many 125 microgram tablets should be given?

4 A patient is prescribed bisoprolol fumarate 10 mg orally. How many 5 mg tablets should be given?

5 A patient is prescribed 300 mg of ranitidine. How many 150 mg tablets should be given?

6 An adult is prescribed 300 mg of sodium valproate oral solution. The bottle label states there are 200 mg in 5 ml. What volume of sodium valproate needs to be administered?

7 An adult is prescribed 250 mg amoxycillin oral suspension. The bottle label states there are 125 mg in 5 ml. What volume of amoxycillin needs to be administered?

8 A child is prescribed 12 mg of furosemide oral solution. The bottle label states there are 8 mg per ml. What volume of furosemide needs to be administered?

9 A patient is prescribed 210 mg of ferrous fumarate syrup. The bottle label states there are 140 mg in 5 ml. What volume of ferrous fumarate needs to be administered?

10 A child is prescribed 62.5 mg of phenoxymethylpenicillin (penicillin V) oral solution. The bottle label states there are 125 mg in 5 ml. What volume of phenoxymethylpenicillin needs to be administered?

11 A patient is prescribed 40 mg of furosemide by injection. The ward stock is 10 mg / ml. What volume should be administered?

12 A patient is prescribed 50 mg of chlorpromazine by injection. The ward stock is 25 mg / ml. What volume should be administered?

13 A patient is prescribed 60 mg of ranitidine by injection. The ward stock is 50 mg / ml. What volume should be administered?

Self-assessment test 4.7: summary test (*continued*)

14 A patient is prescribed 24 mg of morphine by injection. The ward stock is 30 mg / ml. What volume should be administered?

15 A patient is prescribed 175 micrograms of digoxin by injection. The ward stock is 250 microgram / ml. What volume should be administered?

16 A patient is prescribed 1000 ml of intravenous Sodium Chloride 0.9% to run over 7.5 hours. What volume of fluid should run hourly?

17 1000 ml of intravenous Sodium Chloride 0.9% is prescribed to run over 6 hours. Using a standard intravenous infusion set, how many drops per minute are needed to infuse the fluid over the prescribed time?

18 A patient is prescribed 750 ml of intravenous Ringer's solution to run over 3 hours. What volume of fluid should run hourly?

19 A patient is prescribed 750 ml of intravenous Ringer's solution to run over 3 hours. Using a standard intravenous infusion set, how many drops per minute are needed to infuse the fluid over the prescribed time?

20 A patient is prescribed 500 ml of intravenous glucose 5% to run over 4 hours. What volume of fluid should run hourly?

21 A patient is prescribed 500 ml of intravenous glucose 5% to run over 4 hours. Using a standard intravenous infusion set, how many drops per minute are needed to infuse the fluid over the prescribed time?

22 A patient is prescribed 1000 ml of intravenous Ringer's solution to run over 8 hours. What volume of fluid should run hourly?

23 A patient is prescribed 500 ml of intravenous Sodium Chloride 0.9% to run over 6 hours. Using a standard intravenous infusion set, how many drops per minute are needed to infuse the fluid over the prescribed time?

24 A patient is prescribed 500 ml of intravenous Sodium Chloride 0.9% to run over 4.5 hours. What volume of fluid should run hourly?

25 A patient is prescribed 500 ml of intravenous Sodium Chloride 0.9% to run over 2 hours. Using a standard intravenous infusion set, how many drops per minute are needed to infuse the fluid over the prescribed time?

26 A patient is prescribed 5 micrograms of digoxin per kilogram of body weight. If the patient weighs 76 kg, what amount of digoxin needs to be given?

Self-assessment test 4.7: summary test (*continued*)

27 A patient is prescribed an injection of midazolam intramuscularly at 80 micrograms per kilogram of body weight. If the patient weighs 75 kg, what amount of midazolam needs to be given?

28 A patient is prescribed enoxaparin at 1.5 mg (150 units) per kilogram of body weight. If the patient weighs 70 kg, what amount of enoxaparin needs to be given?

29 A nine-month-old baby weighs 8.5 kg and is prescribed morphine 200 micrograms per kilogram of body weight. What amount of morphine needs to be administered?

30 A patient is prescribed 5 mg of gentamicin per kilogram of body weight per day. If the patient weighs 84 kg, what is the total daily amount of gentamicin to be given?

31 A patient is prescribed an intravenous infusion of aminophylline 500 micrograms per kilogram per hour. If the patient weighs 74 kg, what amount of aminophylline should be administered per hour?

32 A child weighing 32 kg is prescribed dexamethasone 300 micrograms per kg of body weight daily. What is the total amount of dexamethasone given over a three-day course?

33 A patient weighing 68 kg is prescribed atenolol 150 micrograms per kg over 20 minutes. How much atenolol will be given?

34 A patient is prescribed dobutamine 5 micrograms per kg per minute. If the patient weighs 75 kg:

    a   **How much dobutamine is administered each minute?**

    b   **How much dobutamine is administered over the period of one hour?**

KEY POINTS TO TAKE AWAY FROM THIS CHAPTER

- Calculating a drug dose is one part of a series of checks to increase patient safety.
- When using the WIG equation, SI units have to be the same, so convert if necessary.
- Calculations involving drugs to be injected, given via a volumetric pump or syringe driver, are classed as complex and must be done by two nurses.

05

OTHER CLINICAL CALCULATIONS

THIS CHAPTER:

- focuses on the application of numeracy skills other than drug calculations, in clinical practice

- outlines the importance of understanding the 24-hour clock

- explores the use of numbers in pressure ulcer risk assessment calculators

- discusses the use of the National Early Warning Score (NEWS2)

- describes the importance of understanding the measurement of pH

- applies numeracy skills to patient hydration and nutrition.

5.1 Introduction

Registered nurses need to be numerate to meet the needs of people in their care. The NMC (2018) indicates that numeracy skills are part of 'Being an accountable professional' (Platform 1), 'Assessing needs and planning care' (Platform 3) and 'Providing and evaluating care' (Platform 4), as well as being integral to many of the nursing procedures outlined in Annexe B of *Future Nurse: standards of proficiency for registered nurses*.

The organisation of care and specifically the measurement, documentation and interpretation of vital signs as well as the management of patients' nutritional and fluid status all depend on an understanding of the 24-hour clock.

5.2 **The 24-hour clock**

The 24-hour clock is used in clinical practice to avoid confusion between the morning (am) and afternoon and evening times (pm) of the 12-hour clock. Most charts and observation records used in healthcare are based on the 24-hour clock.

When using the 24-hour clock, morning times are similar to those of the 12-hour clock but are written as hours, not o'clock.

8 o'clock or 8 am becomes 0800 hours.

0100 hr = 1 am	0200 hr = 2 am	0300 hr = 3 am
0400 hr = 4 am	0500 hr = 5 am	0600 hr = 6 am
0700 hr = 7 am	0800 hr = 8 am	0900 hr = 9 am
1000 hr = 10 am	1100 hr = 11 am	1200 hr = 12 pm / midday

Minutes are written after the hour, for example 0920 hr replaces twenty past nine and 1035 hr replaces twenty-five to eleven. There are no quarter to, quarter past or half past the hours with the 24-hour clock; these are instead written as, for example, 1345 hr, 1015 hr and 1730 hr, respectively.

Afternoon and evening times continue from 1200 hr:

1300 hr = 1 pm	1400 hr = 2 pm	1500 hr = 3 pm
1600 hr = 4 pm	1700 hr = 5 pm	1800 hr = 6 pm
1900 hr = 7 pm	2000 hr = 8 pm	2100 hr = 9 pm
2200 hr = 10 pm	2300 hr = 11 pm	2400 hr = 12 am / midnight

PRACTICE TIP

Prescription charts sometimes use the 24-hour clock but often use daily events like meal or bedtimes to help patients develop a routine in preparation for discharge.

5.3 **Organisation of care**

The organisation of care starts with patient assessment to help identify care needs. This involves the collection and analysis of a broad range of patient data, some in a numerical form using clinical risk assessment calculators like:

- pressure ulcer risk assessment tools

- National Early Warning Score (NEWS)

- Malnutrition Universal Screening Tool ('MUST' score).

With the possible exception of some aspects of nutritional assessment, the arithmetic involved in the use of clinical risk assessment calculators is usually confined to addition and subtraction.

Pressure ulcer risk assessment tools

There are more than 40 tools that assess the risk of developing pressure ulcers.

- The Norton scale is the oldest.

- The Braden scale is the most investigated and researched.

- The Waterlow scale is the one most widely used in the UK.

These tools are designed to indicate which patients are at a higher risk, but their accuracy depends on several factors.

- Sensitivity: This measures the percentage of those who developed a pressure ulcer who were predicted to be at risk.

- Specificity: This is the percentage of those correctly predicted not to be at risk.

Unfortunately these tools are not highly accurate. They are criticised because this may lead to a waste of resources, in terms of both equipment and staff time, in trying to prevent pressure ulcers in patients who won't get them. Also, they may fail to accurately identify all patients at risk, resulting in the development of pressure ulcers in some patients, discomfort, delayed discharge and additional healthcare costs. Griffiths & Jull (2010) reviewed the research evidence about the accuracy of predicting pressure ulcers using the Norton, Braden and Waterlow scales and found that:

- The Norton scale had an accuracy of between 7.1–38%.

- The Braden scale had an accuracy of between 4.5–100%.

- The Waterlow scale had an accuracy of between 5.3–33%.

Although pressure ulcer risk calculators are far from perfect, guidelines state that they should be used alongside clinical judgement to assess patient risk. They may prevent pressure ulcers simply by drawing attention to the problem – the 'Hawthorne' effect.

EXAMPLE 5.1

Mr James Arnold is a 77-year-old male who has been admitted to the community hospital. His wife died 3 months ago and he is still grieving for her. He is a little unkempt and has recently suffered from a chest infection. You notice that his skin in the risk areas is dry and there is some limitation of his mobility – Mr Arnold can't really be bothered. He is continent. When you check his weight, you calculate that he is obese but he says he isn't eating very well at present as his appetite has decreased and he has no interest in food.

As part of the admission procedure, using the Waterlow scale below:

• calculate Mr Arnold's Waterlow score

and

• identify the severity of risk of developing pressure ulcers.

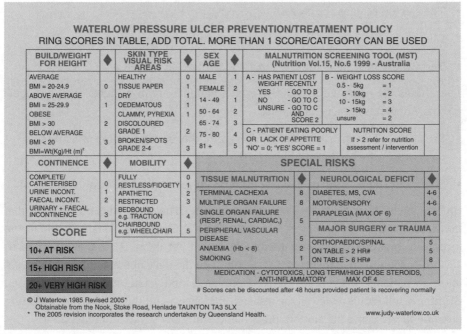

(Chart reproduced by kind permission of Judy Waterlow SRN MBE.)

You need to have noted the following risk factors and scored them:

• Male = 1
• Age 77 = 4
• Dry skin = 1
• Obese = 2
• Loss of appetite = 1
• Continent = 0
• Limited mobility (apathy) = 2

Mr Arnold's total score is 11 which puts him in the 'at risk' category.

EXAMPLE 5.2

Calculate the Waterlow score and risk category for this patient:

Mrs Megan Evans is 76 years old and has been admitted to the stroke rehabilitation unit following a stroke. Her skin looks healthy and she looks well nourished. Mrs Evans says that she is eating properly and has a good appetite. You calculate that her body mass index is 26. She has suffered from type two diabetes for nine years and has smoked for 50 years, although she has made several attempts to stop recently. Following the stroke, her mobility is restricted but she remains continent. The results of blood tests taken on admission show that she is anaemic (haemoglobin 7.6) but apart from this, all observations are normal.

You need to have noted the following risk factors and scored them:

- Female = 2
- Age 76 = 4
- BMI 26 = 1
- Diabetic = 4
- Anaemia = 2
- Smokes = 1
- Restricted mobility = 3

Mrs Evans' total score is 17, which puts her in the 'high risk' category.

> **PRACTICE TIP**
>
> Clinical risk assessment calculators are an important part of patient assessment. The arithmetic involved is basic, but the accuracy of these tools can be limited by design faults. This isn't a reason to stop using them, but a reason to use clinical judgement and experience as well.

The National Early Warning Score 2

The National Early Warning Score (NEWS) is a bedside clinical assessment tool designed to standardise the approach to assessing adult, non-pregnant patients who are acutely ill, and detecting deterioration in such patients (see inside back cover). It aims to ensure that patients are carefully observed, treated by appropriately trained staff and if necessary admitted to a critical care bed. The standardised approach is recommended in order to achieve consistency in the identification and management of acutely ill people across clinical specialities and across the UK.

The NEWS is an aid to clinical assessment and not a substitute for clinical judgement. Any concern about a patient's clinical condition should prompt an urgent clinical review, irrespective of the NEWS.

NEWS tracks six physiological parameters:

- respiration rate

- oxygen saturation

- systolic blood pressure

- pulse rate

- level of consciousness or new confusion (observed change to the patient's mental state such as disorientation or delirium)

- temperature.

A score is allocated to each one of these vital signs. A score of 2 is also added for a patient requiring supplemental oxygen to maintain their prescribed oxygen saturation range. Individual scores are added up to derive the aggregate NEW score for the patient. (See the NEWS charts on the inside back cover.)

There are four trigger levels that prompt a clinical response.

Score	Risk	Response
1–4	Low	Assessed by registered nurse
Score of 3 in any single parameter	Medium	Urgent review by clinician (usually a doctor)
5–6	Medium	Urgent review by clinician (doctor or acute team nurse)
7 +	High	Emergency assessment by clinical team or critical care outreach team

EXAMPLE 5.3

Mrs Jean Winney, age 72 years, has been admitted to the surgical ward following a visit from her GP. She has osteoarthritis and has regularly taken non-steroidal anti-inflammatory drugs for many years. Mrs Winney called the GP because she had suffered with indigestion and abdominal pain for several days, but today felt really unwell. She is quiet, pale and obviously unwell but does manage a weak smile and asks if her daughter has been contacted.

On admission, you take Mrs Winney's vital signs and find the following:

- heart rate 96
- blood pressure 108/62
- temperature 35.9
- respiration rate 18
- oxygen saturation 98%
- level of consciousness: alert.

Using the NEWS chart on the inside back cover, Mrs Winney's score is 3, putting her in the low risk category:
- heart rate 96 = 1
- blood pressure 108/62 = 1 (systolic pressure is the higher / first value)
- temperature 35.9 = 1
- respiration rate 18 = 0
- oxygen saturation 98% = 0
- level of consciousness: alert = 0

EXAMPLE 5.4

Calculate the NEW score and risk category for this patient:

Mr Arnold Joseph, age 82 years, has just been admitted. He has recently had flu and has now developed a chest infection. On arrival he is alert and talking to you, but seems a little breathless.

Mr Joseph's vital signs are:
- heart rate 118
- blood pressure 106/90
- temperature 38.4
- respiration rate 23
- oxygen saturation 94%
- level of consciousness: alert.

Mr Joseph's NEW score is 7, putting him in the 'high risk' category.
- heart rate 118 = 2
- blood pressure 106/90 = 1
- temperature 38.4 = 1
- respiration rate 23 = 2
- oxygen saturation 94% = 1
- level of consciousness: alert = 0

The pH scale

pH is a unit of measurement of the degree of acidity or alkalinity of a solution. The pH scale measures the concentration of hydrogen ions in solution. The measured pH is inversely proportional to the number of hydrogen ions in solution, so as the number of hydrogen ions increases and the solution becomes more acidic, the pH measurement decreases.

0	1	2	3	4	5	6	7	8	9	10	11	12	13	14
Strong acid							Neutral							Highly alkaline

Each whole number on the pH scale represents a tenfold difference in hydrogen ion concentration.

- The pH of the blood is 7.35–7.45 (slightly alkaline).

- The pH of gastric juice is 1.2–3 (strongly acidic).

- The pH of saliva is 6.35–6.85 (slightly acidic).

One aspect of care that relies on the accurate measurement of pH, is the insertion and use of nasogastric feeding tubes. There have been regular reports of feeding tubes becoming misplaced or being incorrectly inserted into the lungs instead of the stomach, leading to patient deaths.

Nasogastric feeding tube position should be confirmed:

- following insertion

- before giving a feed

- before giving medication via the tube

- following any retching, coughing or vomiting

- at least once daily during continuous feeding

- if the exposed tube appears to be longer or displaced.

To check the position of a nasogastric feeding tube, aspirate (gastric fluid) is:

- drawn up the feeding tube using a syringe

- applied onto a pH indicator paper strip.

pH paper strips are graduated at intervals of 0.5 and range from 0–6 or 1–11.

The pH paper must react and show that the fluid has a pH of 5.5 or below. Readings between 1 and 5.5 are a reliable indication that the feeding tube is not in the lungs. If a pH reading of 5.5 or below is not obtained, then this can indicate that the feeding tube has become misplaced and that feeding is unsafe.

ERROR ALERT

Other tests historically used to establish the position of feeding tubes are unsafe. The use of the 'Whoosh test', which involves the use of a stethoscope to hear air bubbling or whooshing when injected down the tube, is not 100% accurate. Testing aspirate for acidity using blue litmus paper, which acids turn red, is flawed as slightly acidic readings have been identified from the tracheo-bronchial secretions of patients.

5.4 **Hydration**

Various nutrients are required by the body including:

- proteins

- fats

- carbohydrates

- fibre

- vitamins

- minerals

- water.

Water is the most common molecule in the body. It plays a key role as the most abundant solvent carrying other nutrients and waste and in the regulation of body temperature.

Water accounts for approximately:

- 60% of the body weight of an adult male

- 50–70% of the body weight in women and children.

Individuals:

- with lower levels of body fat (like children) will have a higher volume of body water

- with larger amounts of body fat (like women or people who are obese) will have a lower volume of water.

> **PRACTICE TIP**
>
> When calculating a patient's fluid balance, it is important to appreciate that individuals do vary. The calculations that you perform need to be accurate but don't lose sight of your patient; numbers might be standardised, but patients are unique.

The management of a patient's hydration involves two processes:

- the measurement of fluid input and output, and

- the calculation of fluid balance.

The measurement of fluid intake and output is a common feature of many practice settings. Although performed frequently, it is important to remember the reasons for monitoring a patient's fluid balance to help ensure that it is performed accurately, and not treated as routine. The procedure is aimed at helping to identify those patients who are dehydrated and those who are at risk of dehydration.

In healthy individuals:

- The amount of fluid consumed is equal to the amount of fluid lost by the body.

- Excess water, wastes and electrolytes are excreted through the kidneys and in the faeces.

- Some water and salt are lost via the skin and respiratory tract.

- Two to three litres of fluid intake daily is considered adequate (in adults).

PRACTICE TIP

Inadequate hydration is a known patient safety issue and a common problem in hospitals. This can rapidly lead to dehydration, a fall in blood pressure, a weakened pulse volume and a rise in the heart rate. Without correction, this can result in renal failure and death. Always make sure that patients have access to fresh drinking water, or are kept hydrated by intravenous or percutaneous endoscopic gastrostomy (peg) routes.

Reasons for measuring and recording fluid intake and output:

- where there is a problem with getting fluids into the body, for example patients who have difficulties in swallowing

- where there may be disruption in the balance of water between the various compartments within the body, for example a patient with hypovolaemic shock

- where there are problems with excreting fluid from the body, as in patients with renal failure.

These categories are not mutually exclusive and can exist together, as in the example of a patient with severe hypovolaemic shock who develops acute renal failure.

Apart from calculation mistakes, there are other factors that will influence the accuracy of fluid balance records:

- insensible loss (fluid loss due to increased sweating or respiration rates)

- estimating a patient's intake if they don't finish a drink

- judging urine output when a patient has suffered from urinary incontinence.

Making allowances for these factors can't be done with any real accuracy but:

- If a patient is pyrexial and sweating or losing extra fluid from increased respirations, take this into account if there is a positive fluid balance over a 24-hour period.

- Don't record a patient's drink on the fluid balance chart until they have finished. Check any left over by measuring; some cups have millilitres marked on the side or you can weigh the cup. Oral fluids weigh approximately 1 gram per ml, but don't forget to subtract the weight of the cup. Alternatively, in your pocket notebook record the volume of three-quarters, half and one-quarter of a cup for future reference.

- Estimating urinary incontinence is difficult but there is considerable difference between dampness of an item of clothing or bedding and something that is soaking wet through. If a patient is drinking normally but their fluid balance chart only records episodes of dampness, then this warrants further investigation to find out if their bladder is emptying properly.

> **PRACTICE TIP**
>
> Use non-numerical information to help validate your calculations. Remember that close relatives may know the patient best and might have noticed changes. Checking the brightness of the eyes, observing if they appear sunken, and noting the smell of a patient's breath can be used to assess for dehydration. Urine colour usually gives an indication of the concentration. Darker urine is more concentrated and paler urine more dilute.

Fluid balance charts

The numeracy skills required to accurately complete fluid balance charts are addition, subtraction and multiplication. While these are some of the basic number skills, it doesn't automatically follow that calculating fluid balance charts is easy. There are many small calculations to be performed. A lapse of concentration or interruption at a critical point may mean starting the calculation all over again, or could lead to an error. Some charts help prevent this by having a 'running total' column.

Fluid balance charts are used to record all fluid intake:

- oral
- intravenous
- tube feeds.

All fluid loss is also recorded:

- urine

- diarrhoea

- via a stoma

- wound drainage

- nasogastric tube aspirate

- vomit.

At the end of the 24-hour period the total fluid intake and output is calculated, and an overall balance arrived at.

- A positive fluid balance is when the amount taken into the body is greater than the amount lost from the body. This might be found when a patient has been admitted in a dehydrated state and is receiving fluid replacement.

- A negative fluid balance is when the loss is greater than intake. This could happen in a patient with heart failure and oedema who has been given diuretic drugs. The excess fluid that has accumulated in the interstitial space is lost from the body, under the influence of the medication.

- Knowledge of the patient's current health problems, drug therapy and renal function are needed to interpret fluid balance. Remember to report any variances in fluid balance to a senior member of staff. They will be able to decide if any variance is significant and requires action.

EXAMPLE 5.5

Mrs Anne Thompson, aged 80 years, has been admitted to a ward in the community hospital following a recent chest infection. This has left her rather frail and unable to look after herself over the last two weeks.
During her first day in hospital Mrs Thompson drinks the following fluids:

Time	Fluid	Volume
1100	Tea	150 ml
1200	Soup	200 ml
1230	Tea	150 ml
1400	Tea	150 ml
1530	Orange juice	100 ml
1600	Tea	150 ml
1700	Custard	100 ml
1800	Tea	150 ml

1900	Tea	150 ml
2100	Chocolate	150 ml
2200	Water	75 ml

She also receives 500 ml of intravenous fluid at 1100 and 500 ml at 1800.
Over the same day, Mrs Thompson's urine output is:

1600	250 ml
1830	380 ml
2200	500 ml

Total input (oral = 1525 ml and intravenous = 1000 ml) = 2525 ml
Total output = 1130 ml
The fluid balance over the 24-hour period = input minus output =
2525 ml − 1130 ml = 1395 ml
Mrs Thompson's input is 1395 ml more than her output, a positive fluid balance. This is likely to be due to her having been dehydrated. Over the last two weeks she may have lost her appetite or been unable to prepare drinks for herself.

ERROR ALERT

Fluid balance charts are a useful record of fluid intake and output, but the accuracy does depend on the staff. Inconsistencies in the interpretation and recording of liquid foods like custard, soup or ice cream can influence accuracy. In many areas of practice, with the exception of neonatal, paediatric and burns units, it is reasonable to think of fluid balance estimation rather than accurate measurement.

Self-assessment test 5.1: calculating fluid balance (1)

This test will help you become familiar with the calculations used when monitoring fluid balance. Answers can be found at the end of the book.

Using the data supplied on the fluid balance chart below, calculate the following:

1 the total oral intake
2 the total intravenous intake
3 the total fluid intake
4 the total urine output
5 the total fluid output

Self-assessment test 5.1: calculating fluid balance (1) (*continued*)

6 the fluid balance for this 24-hour period, indicating whether this is positive or negative.

FLUID BALANCE CHART 1						
PATIENT'S NAME:	Audrey Facer					
DATE OF BIRTH:	09/02/46					
INTAKE				OUTPUT		
TIME	ORAL	I / V	N / G TUBE	URINE	VOMIT / ASPIRATE	DRAIN
0600						
0700				430 ml		
0800						
0900						
1000		500 ml N/Saline		380 ml		
1100	Water 50 ml					
1200	Water 50 ml					
1300	Water 100 ml	500 ml N/Saline		460 ml		
1400	Tea 100 ml					
1500	Tea 150 ml					
1600	Tea 150 ml			520 ml		
1700	Water 100 ml					
1800	Tea 150 ml					
1900	Tea 150 ml			400 ml		
2000	Water 100 ml					
2100	Tea 150 ml					
2200	Water 150 ml			510 ml		
2400						
24-hour totals						

Self-assessment test 5.2: calculating fluid balance (2)

Using the data supplied on the fluid balance chart below, calculate the following:

1 the total oral intake

2 the total intravenous intake

3 the total fluid intake

Self-assessment test 5.2: calculating fluid balance (2) (*continued*)

4 the total urine output

5 the total fluid output

6 the fluid balance for this 24-hour period, indicating whether this is positive or negative.

FLUID BALANCE CHART 2						
PATIENT'S NAME:	Joseph Arnold					
DATE OF BIRTH:	12/07/59					
INTAKE				OUTPUT		
TIME	ORAL	I / V	N / G TUBE	URINE	VOMIT / ASPIRATE	DRAIN
0600		100 ml N/Saline		575 ml		
0700	Tea 100 ml					
0800	Tea 100 ml					150 ml
0900	Orange 200 ml					
1000	Coffee 100 ml	100 ml N/Saline				
1100	Water 150 ml			525 ml		
1200	Water 150 ml					
1300	Orange 100 ml					
1400	Coffee 150 ml	100 ml N/Saline				
1500	Tea 150 ml					
1600	Water 50 ml			600 ml		
1700	Tea 100 ml					50 ml
1800	Water 100 ml	100 ml N/Saline				
1900	Tea 150 ml					
2000	Milk 100 ml					
2100	Chocolate 150 ml					
2200	Water 150 ml	100 ml N/Saline		450 ml		
2400				550 ml		
24-hour totals						

5.5 **Nutritional status**

Adequate nutrition is a prerequisite for the health and well-being of all patients, and good nutrition plays a vital role in recovery from illness.

- In 1859, Florence Nightingale commented that 'Every careful observer of the sick will agree in this that thousands of patients are annually starved in the midst of plenty'.

- 25–34% of patients admitted to hospital are at risk of malnutrition (BAPEN, 2012).

- People who are malnourished have longer hospital stays and a greater number of admissions and re-admissions (BAPEN, 2012).

Providing nutritional support is an enduring problem that has challenged carers throughout recent history. Modern nurses are expected to overcome this challenge. Calculations play a large part in both the assessment and delivery of nutritional care.

Nutrition

Assessing and monitoring nutritional status is part of the organisation of care expected of nurses. Like many other aspects of care, risk assessment is fundamental to this process and begins with the use of a screening tool to:

- identify patients suffering from malnutrition

- identify patients most at risk of malnutrition

- monitor patients already identified as being at risk.

Malnutrition can affect anyone but most at risk are:

- patients with chronic diseases

- the elderly

- people recently discharged from hospital.

The 'Malnutrition Universal Screening Tool' ('MUST') is a universally recognised valid measure of malnutrition in adults and is suitable to use in many clinical settings.

There are five steps in the application of the 'MUST' tool:

- the measurement of height and weight to calculate a body mass index (BMI)

- identifying and calculating unplanned weight loss

- establishing the effect of acute disease

- addition of the individual scores and calculation of the overall risk of malnutrition

- planning and implementation of care to meet identified deficits.

The application of the 'MUST' tool is supported by a comprehensive guide and explanatory booklet, which can be accessed at www.bapen.org.uk. The screening tool provides a BMI chart as well as details used to calculate a weight loss score.

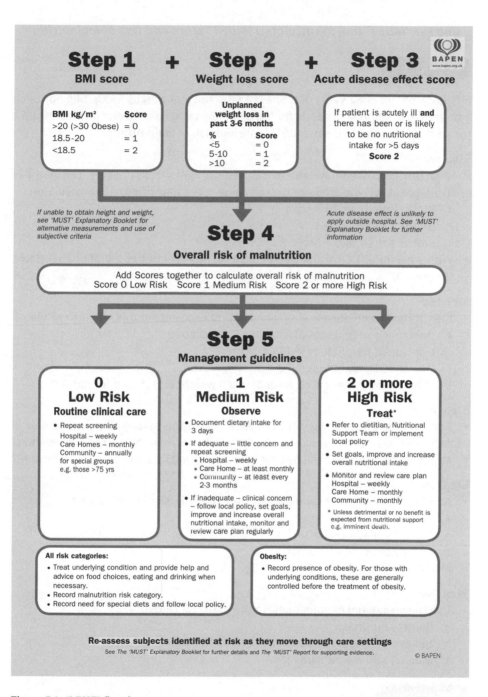

Figure 5.1. *'MUST' flowchart.*

Using the 'MUST' tool to calculate a 'MUST' score and risk of malnutrition

EXAMPLE 5.6

Mrs Rose Wright is 82 years old. She is 1.68 m tall and weighs 59 kg. She has been admitted to hospital with severe flu-like symptoms and has had no nutritional intake for six days. To calculate her 'MUST' score and risk of malnutrition:

Step one
- Measure height and weight to calculate a BMI ('MUST' score calculator is available at: www.bapen.org.uk/screening-for-malnutrition/must-calculator)
  - BMI greater than 20 = score 0
  - BMI 18.5–20 = score 1
  - BMI less than 18.5 = score 2
- With a height of 1.68 m and weight of 59 kg, Mrs Wright has a BMI of 20.9. Score for this = 0

Step two
- Identify and calculate any unplanned weight loss and put this into the calculator.
  - Unplanned weight loss of less than 5% = score 0
  - Unplanned weight loss 5–10% = score 1
  - Unplanned weight loss more than 10% = score 2
- Mrs Wright has experienced no unplanned weight loss. Score for this = 0

Step three
- Consider the effect of any acute disease, where the person has been acutely ill and there has been or is likely to be no nutritional input for more than five days.
- Mrs Wright is acutely ill and has not been able to eat for six days. Score for this = 2

Step four
- Add the scores together and calculate the overall risk of malnutrition.
  - Score 0 = Low risk
  - Score 1 = Medium risk
  - Score 2 or more = High risk
- Mrs Wright's score = 0 + 0 + 2 = 2 High risk

Step five
- Use the management guidelines for the High risk category:
  - Refer to dietitian.
  - Set goals, improve and increase overall nutritional intake.
  - Monitor and review care plan.

EXAMPLE 5.7

Mr Edward Doyle is 48 years old. He is 1.74 m tall and weighs 52 kg. He is an alcoholic and has been admitted from clinic in an unkempt state. Since his last outpatient appointment two months ago, he has lost 8% of body weight. To calculate Mr Doyle's 'MUST' score and risk of malnutrition:

Step one

- Measure height and weight to calculate a BMI ('MUST' score calculator is available at: www.bapen.org.uk/screening-for-malnutrition/must-calculator)
  - BMI greater than 20 = score 0
  - BMI 18.5–20 = score 1
  - BMI less than 18.5 = score 2
- With a height of 1.74 m and weight of 52 kg, Mr Doyle has a BMI of 17.2. Score for this = 2

Step two

- Identify and calculate any unplanned weight loss and put this into the calculator.
  - Unplanned weight loss of less than 5% = score 0
  - Unplanned weight loss 5–10% = score 1
  - Unplanned weight loss more than 10% = score 2
- Mr Doyle has unintentionally lost 8% of his body weight. Score for this = 1

Step three

- Consider the effect of any acute disease, where the person has been acutely ill and there has been or is likely to be no nutritional input for more than five days.
- Mr Doyle is not acutely ill and has been able to eat. Score for this = 0

Step four

- Add the scores together and calculate the overall risk of malnutrition.
  - Score 0 = Low risk
  - Score 1 = Medium risk
  - Score 2 or more = High risk
- Mr Doyle's score = 2 + 1 + 0 = 3 High risk

Step five

- Use the management guidelines for the High risk category:
  - Refer to dietitian.
  - Set goals, improve and increase overall nutritional intake.
  - Monitor and review care plan.

PRACTICE TIP

The BMI charts also convert metric measurements for weight and height into imperial measures, useful for the many patients who still want to know their height in feet and inches and weight in stones and pounds. *Appendix 6* of this book also contains weight and height conversion charts.

The first two steps in calculating a 'MUST' score involve measurements and calculations, but the BMI and weight loss data sheets included in the 'MUST' pack reduce the need for anything overly complicated. If you need to calculate a BMI manually, the formula is below.

5.6 Weight

Calculating a BMI

The BMI is a reliable measure of the relationship between weight and height in adults.

The equation used to calculate a BMI is: $BMI = \dfrac{Weight\ (kg)}{Height\ (m)^2}$

The unit of measurement for a BMI is kg/m^2, although this is frequently omitted and the BMI stated as a figure.

EXAMPLE 5.8

If a patient weighed 74 kg and was 1.71 m tall, the BMI would be calculated as:

$$\frac{74}{1.71 \times 1.71} = \frac{74}{2.9241} = 25.3\,kg/m^2$$

Using the BMI table below, a BMI of 25.3 puts the patient just into the 'overweight' category.

BMI (kg/m²)	Weight status
Below 18.5	Underweight
18.5 – 24.9	Normal
25 – 29.9	Overweight
30 – 39.9	Obese
Above 40	Very obese

EXAMPLE 5.9

If a patient weighed 85 kg and was 1.68 m tall, the BMI would be calculated as:

$$\frac{85}{1.68 \times 1.68} = \frac{85}{2.8224} = 30.1\,kg/m^2$$

Using the BMI table above, a BMI of 30.1 puts the patient just into the 'obese' category.

ERROR ALERT

BMI needs to be used with caution in older adults. It is not sensitive to the loss of height and muscle mass that can occur in later life.

PRACTICE TIP

If a patient cannot stand or get out of bed, and there is no recent reliable record of their weight, use the 'mid upper arm circumference' (MUAC) as an estimation of BMI.

Measure around the upper arm exactly half way between the bony tip of the shoulder (the uppermost part of the scapula called the acromion), and the bony point of the elbow (the olecranon process at the proximal end of the ulna) in centimetres.

- A MUAC less than 23.5 cm indicates that the BMI is likely to be less than 20 kg/m^2.
- A MUAC greater than 30 cm suggests a BMI of more than 30 kg/m^2.

Self-assessment test 5.3: calculating BMI

The recap questions below will help to consolidate your learning about calculating BMI. Answers can be found at the end of the book.

Attempt the following BMI calculations using the equation:

$$BMI = \frac{\text{Weight (kg)}}{\text{Height (m)}^2}$$

1 A male patient is 1.85 m tall and weighs 96.5 kg. Calculate his BMI.

2 A female patient is 1.69 m tall and weighs 59 kg. Calculate her BMI.

3 A female patient is 1.54 m tall and weighs 47.2 kg. Calculate her BMI.

4 A male patient is 1.77 m tall and weighs 77.6 kg. Calculate his BMI.

5 A male patient is 1.84 m tall and weighs 90 kg. Calculate his BMI.

6 A female patient is 1.52 m tall and weighs 72 kg. Calculate her BMI and identify her weight status.

7 A male patient is 1.81 m tall and weighs 88 kg. Calculate his BMI and identify his weight status.

Self-assessment test 5.3: calculating BMI (*continued*)

8 A female patient is 1.66 m tall and weighs 68 kg. Calculate her BMI and identify her weight status.

9 A female patient is 1.6 m tall and weighs 63 kg. Calculate her BMI and identify her weight status.

10 A male patient is 1.76 m tall and weighs 89 kg. Calculate his BMI and identify his weight status.

For additional practice, try using the weight and height measurements of family, friends or fellow students.

Calculating weight loss

Unintentional weight loss during the previous three to six months is factored into the 'MUST' score as this may be part of a serious illness.

PERCENTAGE WEIGHT LOSS OVER 3–6 MONTHS	INDICATES
5–10%	Under-nutrition
10–20%	Nutritional support needed
20% plus	Serious nutritional problems

The equation used to calculate loss of body weight as a percentage is:

$$\text{Percentage weight loss} = \frac{(\text{usual weight kg} - \text{actual weight kg})}{\text{usual weight kg}} \times 100$$

This calculation does depend on the patient having monitored their weight and being able to remember the details at a stressful time. They may be preoccupied with concerns about their health, or anxious because of hospital admission.

EXAMPLE 5.10

Mrs Trish Booker has chronic obstructive pulmonary disease and has taken several courses of antibiotics over the last 10 weeks. She has noticed that her appetite has decreased and that she has lost weight. Before her last hospital admission three months ago, she weighed 58 kg but this has fallen to 53 kg.

To calculate Mrs Booker's weight loss, use the formula:

$$\text{Percentage weight loss} = \frac{(\text{usual weight kg} - \text{actual weight kg})}{\text{usual weight kg}} \times 100$$

Mrs Booker's usual weight = 58 kg and actual weight = 53 kg

So   Percentage weight loss = $\dfrac{(58\,kg - 53\,kg)}{58\,kg} \times 100$

$= \dfrac{5}{58} \times 100 = 0.086 \times 100 = 8.6$

So Mrs Booker has lost 8.6% of her body weight.

EXAMPLE 5.11

Mrs Linda Reid is waiting for the removal of her gall bladder and has noticed a change in her appetite over the last four months. When she first visited her GP about her gall bladder problem, she weighed 66 kg, but now four months later, this has fallen to 59 kg.

To calculate Mrs Reid's weight loss, use the formula:

Percentage weight loss $= \dfrac{(usual\ weight\ kg - actual\ weight\ kg)}{usual\ weight\ kg} \times 100$

Mrs Reid's usual weight = 66 kg and actual weight = 59 kg

So   Percentage weight loss $= \dfrac{(66\,kg - 59\,kg)}{66\,kg} \times 100$

$= \dfrac{7}{66} \times 100 = 0.106 \times 100 = 10.6$

So Mrs Reid has lost 10.6% of her body weight.

Self-assessment test 5.4: 'MUST' score risk calculations

The questions below will help to consolidate your learning about calculating the level of risk using the 'MUST' tool and include weight loss calculations. Answers can be found at the end of the book.

1 A female patient is 1.62 m tall and weighs 78 kg. Her appetite has decreased since the death of her partner four months ago. She has lost 4 kg over the last two months and has not eaten during the last week. Using the 'MUST' tool, calculate her level of risk.

2 A male patient is 1.74 m tall and weighs 62 kg. He has a raised body temperature, a chest infection, and has eaten very little over the last couple of days. During the last three months, he has noticed that his weight has decreased from 67 kg, without dieting. Using the 'MUST' tool, calculate his level of risk.

Self-assessment test 5.4: 'MUST' score risk calculations (*continued*)

3   A female patient is 1.66 m tall and weighs 56 kg. She is able to eat and drink normally, but over the last three months has unintentionally lost 6 kg. Using the 'MUST' tool, calculate her level of risk.

4   A male patient is 1.8 m tall and weighs 67 kg. He is admitted with a history of becoming increasingly frail following a bout of influenza approximately six weeks ago and has lost 5.5 kg of weight. Using the 'MUST' tool, calculate his level of risk.

5   A female patient is 1.6 m tall and weighs 51 kg. She is able to eat and drink, but over the last four months has unintentionally lost 4.5 kg. Using the 'MUST' tool, calculate her level of risk.

6   A male patient is 1.78 m tall and weighs 72 kg. He has intentionally lost 7 kg of weight over the last eight months. He has recently returned from a trip abroad and suspects he may have suffered with food poisoning while he was away. He has not eaten properly for the last six days. Using the 'MUST' tool, calculate his level of risk.

7   A female patient is 1.65 m tall and weighs 84 kg. She has been admitted with an exacerbation of chronic obstructive pulmonary disease. She has noticed a reduction in her appetite but is able to eat and drink. Using the 'MUST' tool, calculate her level of risk.

8   A male patient is 1.72 m tall and weighs 62 kg. He has become increasingly frail over recent months. There is a suspicion that he has an underlying serious illness, yet to be identified. He may have lost weight over the last few weeks as his clothes seem rather baggy and over-sized. He has not managed to eat anything more than a few mouthfuls of porridge over the last six days. Using the 'MUST' tool, calculate his level of risk.

9   A female patient is 1.55 m tall and weighs 71 kg. She has been admitted with a chest infection and suffered a slight cerebrovascular accident two months ago. Her appetite isn't as good as usual, but she is able to eat and drink. Using the 'MUST' tool, calculate her level of risk.

10 A male patient is 1.73 m tall and weighs 71 kg. He has been admitted following a fractured hip and has developed pneumonia. He has eaten very little over the last three days. Using the 'MUST' tool, calculate his level of risk.

Ideal body weight

A person's ideal body weight can be useful as it is an indicator of under- or over-nutrition. It can be used to set targets for weight gain or loss.

To calculate the ideal body weight:

- Women: 45.5 kg (100 lb) for the first 1.52 m (5 ft) of height, adding an extra 2.3 kg (5 lb) per additional 2.5 cm (1 inch).

- Men: 48 kg (106 lb) for the first 1.52 m (5 ft) of height, adding an extra 2.5 kg (6 lb) per additional 2.5 cm (1 inch).

The formulae for calculating ideal body weight date from a time when imperial, rather than metric units of measurement were routinely used. They are included here because many people still think of their height and weight in terms of these units.

The patient's body weight should be within 10 % of the calculated ideal body weight.

Self-assessment test 5.5: ideal body weight calculations

The questions below will help to gain some practice in calculating ideal body weight. Answers can be found at the end of the book.

Calculate the ideal body weight for the following.

1 A male who is 1.67 m tall.

2 A female who is 1.545 m tall.

3 A male who is 1.7 m tall.

4 A female who is 1.68 m tall.

5 A male who is 1.87 m tall.

6 A female who is 1.6 m tall.

7 A male who is 1.77 m tall.

8 A female who is 1.62 m tall.

9 A male who is 1.72 m tall.

10 A female who is 1.57 m tall.

KEY POINTS TO TAKE AWAY FROM THIS CHAPTER

- The 24-hour clock is the standard way of recording time in healthcare so if you aren't fluent with its use, practise for proficiency and safety.
- Assessing patients' needs involves the use of risk assessment calculators. An understanding of how these are designed helps to appreciate why they are a useful adjunct to care decisions, but no replacement for clinical judgement.
- Hydration and nutrition are important components of patient care that demand good calculation skills on a daily basis.

06

SELF-ASSESSMENT TESTS

What this chapter covers

This chapter provides you with three types of tests to help you revise your learning or to help you prepare for a drug calculation test. The first group of tests (tests 6.1 to 6.3) are about SI units and the second group (tests 6.4 to 6.6) are about drug calculations. Tests 6.7 to 6.10 cover all aspects of medicine administration, SI units, drug calculations, the accuracy of measurement and also test your understanding of medication administration records. Answers can be found at the end of the book.

There are lots of apps that provide more practice if you need it, and your university might subscribe to one such as www.safemedicate.com. The RCN also has a free online resource called Safety in Numbers, available at www.rcn.org.uk/clinical-topics/safety-in-numbers.

Test 6.1: working in SI units (1)

Convert the following to micrograms:

1 0.025 mg =

2 0.601 mg =

3 0.909 mg =

4 1.005 mg =

5 1.2 mg =

Convert the following to millilitres:

6 0.25 L =

7 0.905 L =

8 0.02 L =

9   0.3 L =

10 0.075 L =

Convert the following to milligrams:

11 1 microgram =

12 1 kg =

13 500 micrograms =

14 1.2 g =

15 75 micrograms =

Calculate the following (and present the result in the most appropriate units):

16 750 micrograms – 0.25 mg =

17 5 micrograms + 0.05 mg =

18 1.029 mg – 290 micrograms =

19 1.1 g + 10 mg =

20 0.75 g – 500 mg =

Test 6.2: working in SI units (2)

Convert the following to micrograms:

1 0.0056 mg =

2 1.01 mg =

3 2 mg =

4 1 g =

5 3.005 mg =

Convert the following to millilitres:

6 0.05 L =

7 1.002 L =

8 1.6 L =

9 0.009 L =

10 0.106 L =

Convert the following to milligrams:

11 1.5 g =

12 25 micrograms =

13 5 micrograms =

14 2.01 g =

15 $0.032 \text{g} =$

Calculate the following (and present the result in the most appropriate units):

16 $16 \text{micrograms} + 0.999 \text{mg} =$

17 $1.002 \text{micrograms} - 0.02 \text{mg} =$

18 $1 \text{g} - 5 \text{mg} =$

19 $995 \text{mg} + 0.005 \text{g} =$

20 $890 \text{mg} + 0.111 \text{g} =$

Test 6.3: working in SI units (3)

Convert the following to micrograms:

1 $0.35 \text{mg} =$

2 $3 \text{mg} =$

3 $2.002 \text{mg} =$

4 $0.006 \text{mg} =$

5 $0.75 \text{g} =$

Convert the following to millilitres:

6 $0.75 \text{L} =$

7 $1.03 \text{L} =$

8 $0.005 \text{L} =$

9 $0.04 \text{L} =$

10 $2.02 \text{L} =$

Convert the following to milligrams:

11 $2.2 \text{g} =$

12 $6 \text{micrograms} =$

13 $0.02 \text{g} =$

14 $65 \text{micrograms} =$

15 $0.8 \text{kg} =$

Calculate the following (and present the results in the most appropriate units):

16 $0.9 \text{g} - 8 \text{mg} =$

17 $0.08 \text{mg} + 15 \text{micrograms} =$

18 $1.2 \text{mg} - 400 \text{micrograms} =$

19 $0.75 \text{mg} + 300 \text{micrograms} =$

20 $75 \text{mg} + 0.005 \text{g} =$

Test 6.4: calculating drug doses (1)

Tablets

1   A patient is prescribed 90 mg of a drug. How many 30 mg tablets should be given?

2   A patient is prescribed 45 mg of a drug. How many 30 mg tablets should be given?

3   A patient is prescribed 125 mg of a drug. How many 25 mg tablets should be given?

4   A patient is prescribed 50 mg of a drug. How many 100 mg tablets should be given?

5   A patient is prescribed 45 mg of a drug. How many 15 mg tablets should be given?

6   A patient is prescribed 750 mg of a drug. How many 300 mg tablets should be given?

7   A patient is prescribed 25 mg of a drug. How many 12.5 mg tablets should be given?

8   A patient is prescribed 500 mg of a drug. How many 250 mg tablets should be given?

9   A patient is prescribed 30 micrograms of a drug. How many 5 microgram tablets should be given?

10 A patient is prescribed 1.5 g of a drug. How many 500 mg tablets should be given?

Liquid medicines

11 A patient is prescribed 20 mg of a liquid medicine. The label states that there are 40 mg of the drug in 10 ml. What volume of medicine should be given?

12 A liquid medicine contains 240 mg in 5 ml. How many milligrams are in 24 ml?

13 A liquid medicine contains 60 mg in 5 ml. How many milligrams are in 15 ml?

14 A liquid medicine contains 240 mg in 5 ml. How many milligrams are in 11 ml?

15 A liquid medicine contains 120 mg in 8 ml. How many milligrams are in 15 ml?

Injections

16 A patient is prescribed 160 mg of a drug by injection. The ward stock is 80 mg/ml. What volume should be drawn up in the syringe?

17 A patient is prescribed 75 mg of a drug by injection. The ward stock is 50 mg/ml. What volume should be drawn up in the syringe?

18 A patient is prescribed 110 mg of a drug by injection. The ward stock is 50 mg in 2 ml. What volume should be drawn up in the syringe?

19 A patient is prescribed 90 mg of a drug by injection. The ward stock is 60 mg in 2 ml. What volume should be drawn up in the syringe?

20 A patient is prescribed 75 mg of a drug by injection. The ward stock is 25 mg/ml. What volume should be drawn up in the syringe?

Test 6.5: calculating drug doses (2)

Tablets

1 A patient is prescribed 150 mg of a drug. How many 30 mg tablets should be given?

2 A patient is prescribed 500 mg of a drug. How many 1 g tablets should be given?

3 A patient is prescribed 15 mg of a drug. How many 6 mg tablets should be given?

4 A patient is prescribed 150 mg of a drug. How many 50 mg tablets should be given?

5 A patient is prescribed 60 mg of a drug. How many 120 mg tablets should be given?

6 A patient is prescribed 1.5 g of a drug. How many 750 mg tablets should be given?

7 A patient is prescribed 1 g of a drug. How many 250 mg tablets should be given?

8 A patient is prescribed 750 micrograms of a drug. How many 250 microgram tablets should be given?

9 A patient is prescribed 1.2 g of a drug. How many 300 mg tablets should be given?

10 A patient is prescribed 450 mg of a drug. How many 300 mg tablets should be given?

Liquid medicines

11 A patient is prescribed 60 mg of a liquid medicine. The label states that there are 20 mg of the drug in 5 ml. What volume of medicine should be given?

12 A liquid medicine contains 60 mg in 5 ml. How many milligrams are in 17 ml?

13 A liquid medicine contains 120 mg in 8 ml. How many milligrams are in 18 ml?

14 A liquid medicine contains 60 mg in 5 ml. How many milligrams are in 25 ml?

15 A liquid medicine contains 240 mg in 5 ml. How many milligrams are in 18 ml?

Injections

16 A patient is prescribed 120 mg of a drug by injection. The ward stock is 40 mg / ml. What volume should be drawn up in the syringe?

17 A patient is prescribed 60 mg of a drug by injection. The ward stock is 120 mg / ml. What volume should be drawn up in the syringe?

18 A patient is prescribed 50 mg of a drug by injection. The ward stock is 40 mg in 2 ml. What volume should be drawn up in the syringe?

19 A patient is prescribed 8 mg of a drug by injection. The ward stock is 10 mg in 2 ml. What volume should be drawn up in the syringe?

20 A patient is prescribed 125 mg of a drug by injection. The ward stock is 50 mg / ml. What volume should be drawn up in the syringe?

Test 6.6: calculating drug doses (3)

Tablets

1 A patient is prescribed 25 mg of a drug. How many 12.5 mg tablets should be given?

2 A patient is prescribed 60 mg of a drug. How many 15 mg tablets should be given?

3 A patient is prescribed 1.2 g of a drug. How many 400 mg tablets should be given?

4 A patient is prescribed 75 micrograms of a drug. How many 25 microgram tablets should be given?

5 A patient is prescribed 140 mg of a drug. How many 70 mg tablets should be given?

6 A patient is prescribed 12 micrograms of a drug. How many 3 microgram tablets should be given?

7 A patient is prescribed 450 mg of a drug. How many 150 mg tablets should be given?

8 A patient is prescribed 15 mg of a drug. How many 7.5 mg tablets should be given?

9 A patient is prescribed 16 mg of a drug. How many 4 mg tablets should be given?

10 A patient is prescribed 45 mg of a drug. How many 15 mg tablets should be given?

Liquid medicines

11 A patient is prescribed 40 mg of a liquid medicine. The label states that there are 80 mg of the drug in 10 ml. What volume of medicine should be given?

12 A patient is prescribed 60 mg of a liquid medicine. The label states that there are 3 mg of the drug in 1 ml. What volume of medicine should be given?

13 A liquid medicine contains 100 mg in 5 ml. How many milligrams are in 17 ml?

14 A liquid medicine contains 80 mg in 4 ml. How many milligrams are in 10 ml?

15 A liquid medicine contains 240 mg in 5 ml. How many milligrams are in 3 ml?

Injections

16 A patient is prescribed 25 mg of a drug by injection. The ward stock is 100 mg in 2 ml. What volume should be drawn up in the syringe?

17 A patient is prescribed 60 mg of a drug by injection. The ward stock is 40 mg/ml. What volume should be drawn up in the syringe?

18 A patient is prescribed 4 mg of a drug by injection. The ward stock is 16 mg in 2 ml. What volume should be drawn up in the syringe?

19 A patient is prescribed 12.5 mg of a drug by injection. The ward stock is 5 mg/ml. What volume should be drawn up in the syringe?

20 A patient is prescribed 5 mg of a drug by injection. The ward stock is 4 mg/ml. What volume should be drawn up in the syringe?

Test 6.7

Conversions

Convert the following to micrograms:

1 0.009 mg =

2 0.057 mg =

Convert the following to millilitres:

3 0.248 L =

4 0.002 L =

Convert the following to milligrams:

5 6 micrograms =

6 2.3 g =

Calculations

7 A patient is prescribed 450 mg of a drug. How many 150 mg tablets should be given?

8 A patient is prescribed 1 mg of a drug. How many 500 microgram tablets should be given?

9 A patient is prescribed 120 mg of a liquid medicine. The label states that there are 20 mg of the drug in 5 ml. What volume of medicine should be given?

10 A patient is prescribed 220 mg of a drug by injection. The ward stock is 100 mg/ml. What volume should be drawn up in the syringe?

Measurement

Syringes are available in several sizes. Drawing up medication in a syringe to accurately reflect the prescription is a common task in clinical practice. Reading the volume contained in the syringe is a prerequisite to accuracy.

SYRINGE SIZE	NUMBER OF GRADUATIONS	VOLUME OF EACH GRADUATION
1 ml	20	0.05 ml
2 ml	20	0.1 ml
5 ml	25	0.2 ml

What volume do the following syringes show?

11

12

13

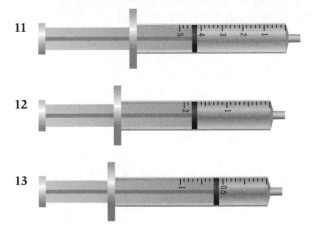

14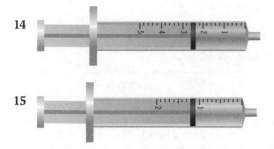

15

Medicine pots are commonly used for the administration of oral solutions. When measuring liquids in a pot, read the lower meniscus line as the liquid may rise slightly against the medicine pot wall.

What volume do the following medicine pots show?

16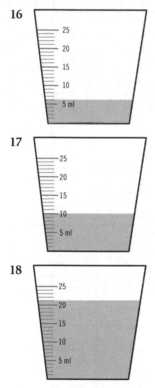

17

18

Medication administration

The following questions relate to the medication administration record below. Advice on reading these can be found in *Appendix 3*.

NAME OF PATIENT:		Chloe Edwards			DOB:		22/05/60		
ROUTE	oral	MEDICATION:		Propranolol	ALLERGIES:		Penicillin		
DATE	20/10				DR'S SIGNATURE:		Dr E Wright		
	DOSE	20/10	21/10	22/10	23/10	24/10	25/10	26/10	27/10
MORNING	80 mg	HD	HD	HD					
MIDDAY									
EVENING	80 mg	RT	RT						
BEDTIME									

ROUTE	oral	MEDICATION:		Furosemide	ALLERGIES:		Penicillin		
DATE	20/10				DR'S SIGNATURE:		Dr E Wright		
	DOSE	20/10	21/10	22/10	23/10	24/10	25/10	26/10	27/10
MORNING	40 mg	HD	HD	HD					
MIDDAY									
EVENING									
BEDTIME									

ROUTE	oral	MEDICATION:		Prednisolone (soluble)	ALLERGIES:		Penicillin		
DATE	20/10				DR'S SIGNATURE:		Dr E Wright		
	DOSE	20/10	21/10	22/10	23/10	24/10	25/10	26/10	27/10
MORNING	20 mg	HD	HD	HD					
MIDDAY									
EVENING									
BEDTIME									

19 The patient's next dose of propranolol is to be given on the evening of 21/10.

True / False

20 The patient is allergic to penicillin. True / False

21 The patient's next dose of furosemide is one 40 mg tablet to be given on 23/10. True / False

22 The prescription is for Chloe Evans. True / False

23 The next dose of prednisolone (soluble), due on the morning of 23/10, is five 5 mg tablets. True / False

24 Identify seven errors in the following medication administration record:

NAME OF PATIENT:		Angharad Graham			DOB:		28/07/45		
ROUTE	oral	MEDICATION:		Co-codamol 30/500	ALLERGIES:			Penicillin	
DATE	20/10				DR'S SIGNATURE:				
	DOSE	20/10	21/10	22/10	23/10	24/10	25/10	26/10	27/10
MORNING	two								
MIDDAY	two								
EVENING	two								
BEDTIME	two								

ROUTE	oral	MEDICATION:		Amoxicillin	ALLERGIES:			Penicillin	
DATE					DR'S SIGNATURE:			Dr E Wright	
	DOSE	20/10	21/10	22/10	23/10	24/10	25/10	26/10	27/10
MORNING	250 mg								
MIDDAY									
EVENING									
BEDTIME									

ROUTE		MEDICATION:		Paracetamol	ALLERGIES:			Penicillin	
DATE					DR'S SIGNATURE:			Dr E Wright	
	DOSE	20/10	21/10	22/10	23/10	24/10	25/10	26/10	27/10
MORNING	1 g								
MIDDAY	1 g								
EVENING	1 g								
BEDTIME	1 g								

Test 6.8

Conversions

Convert the following to micrograms:

1 0.306 mg =

2 0.001 mg =

Convert the following to millilitres:

3 0.407 L =

4 2.02 L =

Convert the following to milligrams:

5 600 micrograms =

6 72 micrograms =

Calculations

7 A patient is prescribed 125 mg of a drug. How many 50 mg tablets should be given?

8 A patient is prescribed 1.5 g of a drug. How many 500 mg tablets should be given?

9 A liquid medicine contains 120 mg in 8 ml. How many milligrams are in 22 ml?

10 A patient is prescribed 250 mg of a drug by injection. The ward stock is 1 g in 2 ml. What volume should be drawn up in the syringe?

Measurement

Syringes are available in several sizes. Drawing up medication in a syringe to accurately reflect the prescription is a common task in clinical practice. Reading the volume contained in the syringe is a prerequisite to accuracy.

SYRINGE SIZE	NUMBER OF GRADUATIONS	VOLUME OF EACH GRADUATION
1 ml	20	0.05 ml
2 ml	20	0.1 ml
5 ml	25	0.2 ml

What volume is shown by the following syringes?

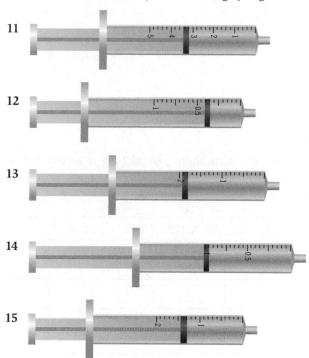

11

12

13

14

15

Medicine pots are commonly used for the administration of oral solutions. When measuring liquids in a pot, read the lower meniscus line as the liquid may rise slightly against the medicine pot wall.

What volume do the following medicine pots show?

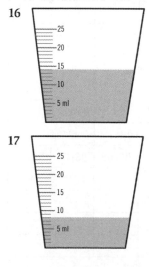

16

17

18

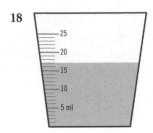

Medication administration

The following questions relate to the medication administration record below. Advice on reading these can be found in *Appendix 3*.

NAME OF PATIENT:	Raymond Owen				DOB:		12/02/52		
ROUTE	oral	MEDICATION:		Phenytoin	ALLERGIES:		None		
DATE	28/07				DR'S SIGNATURE:		Dr E Wright		
	DOSE	28/07	29/07	30/07	31/07	01/08	02/08	03/08	04/08
MORNING	200 mg	PB	PB						
MIDDAY									
EVENING									
BEDTIME									

ROUTE	oral	MEDICATION:		Nitrofurantoin	ALLERGIES:		None		
DATE	28/07				DR'S SIGNATURE:		Dr E Wright		
	DOSE	28/07	29/07	30/07	31/07	01/08	02/08	03/08	04/08
MORNING	50 mg	PB	PB						
MIDDAY	50 mg	PB							
EVENING	50 mg	TC							
BEDTIME	50 mg	SJ							

ROUTE	oral	MEDICATION:		Paracetamol	ALLERGIES:		None		
DATE	28/07				DR'S SIGNATURE:		Dr E Wright		
	DOSE	28/07	29/07	30/07	31/07	01/08	02/08	03/08	04/08
MORNING	1 g	PB	PB						
MIDDAY	1 g	PB							
EVENING	1 g	TC							
BEDTIME	1 g	SJ							

19 The total amount of paracetamol taken over seven days will be 35 g.

True / False

20 The next dose of nitrofurantoin is 100 mg at midday on 29/07.   True / False

21 The prescription is for Raymond Owen.   True / False

22 The next dose of paracetamol, due at midday on 29/07, is two 250 mg tablets.

True / False

23 To complete a seven-day course of nitrofurantoin, there must be another 23 tablets in the bottle.   True / False

24 Identify seven errors in the following medication administration record:

NAME OF PATIENT:				DOB:					
ROUTE	intravenous	MEDICATION:	Phenytoin suspension	ALLERGIES:					
DATE	28/07			DR'S SIGNATURE:	Dr E Wright				
	DOSE	28/07	29/07	30/07	31/07	01/08	02/08	03/08	04/08
MORNING	300 mg								
MIDDAY									
EVENING									
BEDTIME									

ROUTE	oral	MEDICATION:	Digoxin	ALLERGIES:					
DATE				DR'S SIGNATURE:	Dr E Wright				
	DOSE	28/07	29/07	30/07	31/07	01/08	02/08	03/08	04/08
MORNING	250 mg								
MIDDAY									
EVENING									
BEDTIME									

ROUTE	oral	MEDICATION:	Paracetamol	ALLERGIES:					
DATE	28/07			DR'S SIGNATURE:					
	DOSE	28/07	29/07	30/07	31/07	01/08	02/08	03/08	04/08
MORNING	1.5 g								
MIDDAY	1.5 g								
EVENING	1.5 g								
BEDTIME	1.5 g								

Test 6.9

Conversions

Convert the following to micrograms:

1   2.022 mg =

2   0.101 mg =

Convert the following to millilitres:

3   0.082 L =

4   2.01 L =

Convert the following to milligrams:

5   0.053 g =

6   9 micrograms =

Calculations

7   A patient is prescribed 75 mg of a drug. How many 25 mg tablets should be given?

8   A patient is prescribed 250 micrograms of a drug. How many 125 microgram tablets should be given?

9   A liquid medicine contains 60 mg in 5 ml. How many milligrams are in 32 ml?

10   A patient is prescribed 90 mg of a drug by injection. The ward stock is 180 mg in 5 ml. What volume should be drawn up in the syringe?

Measurement

Syringes are available in several sizes. Drawing up medication in a syringe to accurately reflect the prescription is a common task in clinical practice. Reading the volume contained in the syringe is a prerequisite to accuracy.

SYRINGE SIZE	NUMBER OF GRADUATIONS	VOLUME OF EACH GRADUATION
1 ml	20	0.05 ml
2 ml	20	0.1 ml
5 ml	25	0.2 ml

What volume is shown by the following syringes?

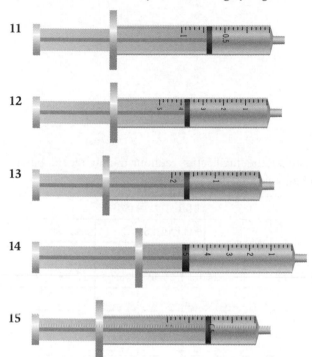

11

12

13

14

15

Medicine pots are commonly used for the administration of oral solutions. When measuring liquids in a pot, read the lower meniscus line as the liquid may rise slightly against the medicine pot wall.

What volume do the following medicine pots show?

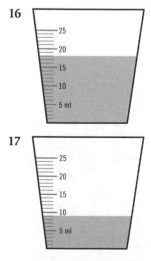

16

17

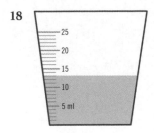

Medication administration

The following questions relate to the medication administration record below. Advice on reading these can be found in *Appendix 3*.

NAME OF PATIENT:	Alan Wood				DOB:		09/12/58		
ROUTE	oral	MEDICATION:		Metformin	ALLERGIES:		Trimethoprim		
DATE	21/09				DR'S SIGNATURE:		Dr E Wright		
	DOSE	21/09	22/09	23/09	24/09	25/09	26/09	27/09	28/09
MORNING	500 mg	SD	SD						
MIDDAY	500 mg	KW	KG						
EVENING	500 mg	ND	ND						
BEDTIME									

ROUTE	oral	MEDICATION:		Atenolol	ALLERGIES:		Trimethoprim		
DATE	21/09				DR'S SIGNATURE:		Dr E Wright		
	DOSE	21/09	22/09	23/09	24/09	25/09	26/09	27/09	28/09
MORNING	50 mg	SD	SD						
MIDDAY									
EVENING	50 mg	ND	ND						
BEDTIME									

ROUTE	oral	MEDICATION:		Omeprazole	ALLERGIES:		Trimethoprim		
DATE	21/09				DR'S SIGNATURE:		Dr E Wright		
	DOSE	21/09	22/09	23/09	24/09	25/09	26/09	27/09	28/09
MORNING	20 mg	SD	SD						
MIDDAY									
EVENING									
BEDTIME									

19 The patient takes 2 g of metformin over each 24-hour period.

True / False

20 The patient is allergic to trimeprazine. True / False

21 The patient's next dose of omeprazole is one 20 mg tablet to be given on 23/09. True / False

22 The prescription is for Alan Wood. True / False

23 Atenolol 15 mg is next due on 23/09. True / False

24 Identify seven errors in the following medication administration record:

NAME OF PATIENT:	Lynne Bedson			DOB:		13/06/32		
ROUTE	oral	MEDICATION:	Digoxin	ALLERGIES:		None known		
DATE	21/09			DR'S SIGNATURE:				
	DOSE	21/09	22/09	23/09	24/09	25/09	26/09	27/09	28/09
MORNING	250 micrograms								
MIDDAY									
EVENING	250 micrograms								
BEDTIME									

ROUTE	oral	MEDICATION:	Simvastatin	ALLERGIES:		None known		
DATE				DR'S SIGNATURE:				
	DOSE	21/09	22/09	23/09	24/09	25/09	26/09	27/09	28/09
MORNING									
MIDDAY									
EVENING									
BEDTIME	400 mg								

ROUTE		MEDICATION:	Furosemide	ALLERGIES:		None known		
DATE	21/09			DR'S SIGNATURE:		Dr E Wright		
	DOSE	21/09	22/09	23/09	24/09	25/09	26/09	27/09	28/09
MORNING									
MIDDAY									
EVENING									
BEDTIME	40 mg								

Test 6.10

Conversions

Convert the following to micrograms:

1 0.275 mg =

2 0.016 mg =

Convert the following to millilitres:

3 0.072 L =

4 0.902 L =

Convert the following to milligrams:

5 1.25 g =

6 35 micrograms =

Calculations

7 A patient is prescribed 225 mg of a drug. How many 75 mg tablets should be given?

8 A patient is prescribed 1.5 mg of a drug. How many 750 microgram tablets should be given?

9 A liquid medicine contains 60 mg in 4 ml. How many milligrams are in 15 ml?

10 A patient is prescribed 120 mg of a drug by injection. The ward stock is 160 mg in 2 ml. What volume should be drawn up in the syringe?

Measurement

Syringes are available in several sizes. Drawing up medication in a syringe to accurately reflect the prescription is a common task in clinical practice. Reading the volume contained in the syringe is a prerequisite to accuracy.

SYRINGE SIZE	NUMBER OF GRADUATIONS	VOLUME OF EACH GRADUATION
1 ml	20	0.05 ml
2 ml	20	0.1 ml
5 ml	25	0.2 ml

What volume do the following syringes show?

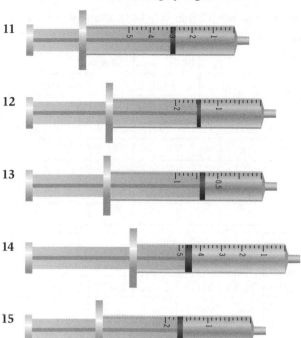

11

12

13

14

15

Medicine pots are commonly used for the administration of oral solutions. When measuring liquids in a pot, read the lower meniscus line as the liquid may rise slightly against the medicine pot wall.

What volume do the following medicine pots show?

16

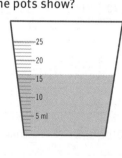

17

18

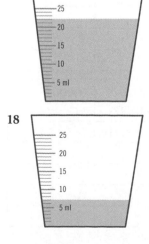

Medication administration

The following questions relate to the medication administration record below. Advice on reading these can be found in *Appendix 3*.

NAME OF PATIENT:		Lily Comrie				DOB:		21/09/58		
ROUTE	oral	MEDICATION:		Bisoprolol		ALLERGIES:		None known		
DATE	20/10					DR'S SIGNATURE:		Dr E Wright		
	DOSE	20/10	21/10	22/10	23/10	24/10	25/10	26/10	27/10	
MORNING	1.25 mg	JD	JD	JD						
MIDDAY										
EVENING										
BEDTIME										

ROUTE	oral	MEDICATION:		Clopidogrel		ALLERGIES:		None known		
DATE	20/10					DR'S SIGNATURE:		Dr E Wright		
	DOSE	20/10	21/10	22/10	23/10	24/10	25/10	26/10	27/10	
MORNING	75 mg	JD	JD	JD						
MIDDAY										
EVENING										
BEDTIME										

ROUTE	oral	MEDICATION:		Irbesartan		ALLERGIES:		None known		
DATE	20/10					DR'S SIGNATURE:		Dr E Wright		
	DOSE	20/10	21/10	22/10	23/10	24/10	25/10	26/10	27/10	
MORNING	300 mg	JD	JD	JD						
MIDDAY										
EVENING										
BEDTIME										

ROUTE	oral	MEDICATION:		Lansoprazole		ALLERGIES:		None known		
DATE	20/10					DR'S SIGNATURE:		Dr E Wright		
	DOSE	20/10	21/10	22/10	23/10	24/10	25/10	26/10	27/10	
MORNING	30 mg	JD	JD	JD						
MIDDAY										
EVENING										
BEDTIME										

19 The patient's next dose of irbesartan is for three 300 mg tablets due on the morning of 23/10. True / False

20 Clopidogrel 50 mg, to be given in the morning, is prescribed daily. True / False

21 The prescription is for Lily Comrie. True / False

22 The patient's next dose of lansoprazole is for 300 mg to be taken on the morning of 23/10. True / False

23 How many milligrams of bisoprolol will be taken over 7 days?

24 How many grams of irbesartan will be taken over 7 days?

25 Identify six errors in the following medication administration record:

NAME OF PATIENT:	Eve Davison				DOB:				
ROUTE		MEDICATION:	Perindopril		ALLERGIES:		None known		
DATE	20/10				DR'S SIGNATURE:		Dr E Wright		
	DOSE	20/10	21/10	22/10	23/10	24/10	25/10	26/10	27/10
MORNING	6 mg								
MIDDAY									
EVENING									
BEDTIME									

ROUTE	oral	MEDICATION:	Amlodipine		ALLERGIES:		None known		
DATE					DR'S SIGNATURE:				
	DOSE	20/10	21/10	22/10	23/10	24/10	25/10	26/10	27/10
MORNING	5 mg								
MIDDAY									
EVENING									
BEDTIME									

ROUTE		MEDICATION:	Omeprazole		ALLERGIES:		None known		
DATE	19/10				DR'S SIGNATURE:		Dr E Wright		
	DOSE	20/10	21/10	22/10	23/10	24/10	25/10	26/10	27/10
MORNING	100 mg								
MIDDAY									
EVENING	100 mg								
BEDTIME									

APPENDIX 1
ADMINISTERING MEDICINES SAFELY

The focus of this book is how to perform calculations accurately. Calculating the correct drug dosage is one of the keystones of safe clinical practice but ensuring patients get the correct dose depends on more than numeracy skills alone. Nurses also need to use their knowledge of individual patients, pharmacology and a safe checking procedure. In addition, nurses need to have a way of checking that what they are about to do seems sensible, some sort of application of common sense.

A safe checking procedure: The '5 Rights'

1. Make sure that you give the drug to the 'right patient' using an identification band or patient photograph check.

2. Make sure it is the 'right drug' by checking the prescription against the label on the medication.

3. Make sure you give the drug by the 'right route', check the prescription.

4. Make sure that you give the drug at the 'right time', check the prescription.

5. Perform the necessary calculations to get the 'right dose'.

Pause before you administer the drug to the patient and ask yourself 'does my answer to the calculation seem reasonable'? Alarm bells should ring if your answer means that you are giving more than four tablets of the same drug or if you need to use more than two ampoules of the drug. Check your calculation with a colleague, it may be correct but better to check before administration than realise a mistake afterwards.

ERROR ALERT

Sometimes the pressure of the clinical environment can lead to nurses not stopping to question a calculation that seems so obviously wrong. Some years ago, two nurses working a night shift on a busy medical ward received a phone call to inform them that a patient was being admitted following an overdose of paracetamol and needed to receive the antidote intravenously.

Usually, this procedure was performed in ITU, but no beds were available. The nurses read the prescription and calculated that forty-five 10 ml ampoules of the drug were needed and then proceeded to inject this into a 500 ml bag of intravenous fluid. In the cold light of day it seems ridiculous that the nurses attempted and managed to draw up forty-five ampoules and inject 450 ml of fluid into a 500 ml bag. It also seems bizarre that although they needed the entire stock of several medical wards to treat one patient, they didn't question this. Predictably and tragically, the patient died.

Pausing before giving the drug and asking 'does my answer to the calculation seem reasonable?' may have led to a significantly different outcome for the patient and the nurses.

APPENDIX 2
ROUTES OF ADMINISTRATION

There are different ways of giving medication to patients. The route identified on the prescription will have been decided upon after considering the following factors:

- **The availability of the route in the clinical situation**

  A patient in shock will absorb drugs given intramuscularly very slowly compared to those given intravenously. A patient may be unable to swallow following a CVA or some types of surgery.

- **The speed and length of action needed**

  Rapid pain relief is essential if a patient is having a heart attack and would be given intravenously. Someone with chronic pain may use patches for a continuous effect.

- **Patient concordance**

  The chosen route should mean that the patient is able to self-medicate unassisted, understands why this is necessary and can act as a partner in their own care.

- **Manual dexterity**

  Does the patient have the strength and co-ordination in their hands to self-medicate? This is an important consideration with some types of inhalers and syringes.

ROUTE (ABBREVIATION)	DESCRIPTION
Buccal	The tablet or liquid is placed inside the mouth between the cheek and gum. Can be used as an alternative to the sublingual route.
Eye drops	Eye drops are instilled into the patient's lower eyelid with their head tilted backwards. The dropper should be vertical and about 2.5 cm from the eye, never touching.
Inhaled (INH)	Drugs can be inhaled into the lungs in an aerosol form intended to act locally within the respiratory system.
Intramuscular (IM)	The drug is injected directly into muscle tissue, commonly the ventrogluteal muscle in adults, when a more rapid absorption is needed.
Intravenous (IV)	Used when an immediate response is needed, the drug is injected directly into a vein so there is no time delay while it is absorbed.
Nasogastric (NG)	The drug is administered via a nasogastric tube.
Nebulised (NEB)	The drug is inhaled into the lungs in a nebulised form intended to act locally within the respiratory system.
Oral (O)	The drug is given by mouth and usually swallowed but in some instances, it can be chewed or sucked.
Percutaneous endoscopic gastrostomy tube (PEG)	The drug is administered via a patient's PEG feed tube, a flexible tube that goes through the abdomen and into the stomach and provides a route for feeding and giving medication.
Rectal (per rectum / PR)	The drug is administered into the rectum as a solution (enema) or small pellet (suppository).
Subcutaneous (SC)	The drug is injected into the fat and connective tissue underneath the dermis at an angle of 45 degrees.
Sublingual (SL)	The drug is placed under the tongue and left to absorb. This route is frequently used for drugs that have an effect on the heart.
Topical (TOP)	Creams and ointments are applied directly to the skin where they are absorbed.
Transdermal	The drug is given by an adhesive 'patch' that releases the medication over a long period of time.
Vaginal (per vagina / PV)	The drug is given in the form of a solid pellet designed to have a local therapeutic action.

The use of some abbreviations is a known source of error. Check with your Drug Policy to identify the permitted abbreviations for where you work.

APPENDIX 3
MEDICATION ADMINISTRATION RECORDS

All documents (such as a prescription or medication administration record) that direct the administration of drugs and medicinal products must be computer generated or written in ink.

Medication administration records must clearly state:

- The name of the patient

- Date of birth

- Generic name of the drug and:

  - The strength of the drug

  - The dose and frequency

    - Dosages must be stated in ml, mg or g. Micrograms must be written in full and not abbreviated

  - Route of administration

  - Minimum dose intervals for drugs taken when needed, e.g. not more than every 6 hours

- The date that the drug is to start

- The weight of the patient if a child or the drug is calculated on body weight

- The height of the patient if the drug is calculated by surface area

- Any allergies that the patient may have and if none, this should be stated.

The medication administration record must be signed and dated by the prescriber.

ERROR ALERT

Although patient records may contain crucial information, nurses still have to act on it.

A patient was admitted to a Plymouth hospital in 2012 following a fall. The ambulance crew and A&E department were told about his penicillin allergy, medical records clearly documented this and the patient wore a red wristband to alert staff. Yet the patient died three days after being given penicillin.

APPENDIX 4
DRUG GLOSSARY

Amantadine
An antiviral drug that is also used in the control of some symptoms of Parkinson's disease

Amiloride
A potassium sparing diuretic drug that can be used to control hypertension and congestive heart failure

Amlodipine
A calcium-channel blocking drug used to treat high blood pressure

Amoxycillin
A broad-based, semi-synthetic penicillin drug often used to treat respiratory infections

Ampicillin
A broad spectrum semi-synthetic penicillin often used to treat respiratory infections; it has a similar action to other penicillins but is also effective against some Gram-negative pathogens

Atenolol
A beta-adrenoceptor blocking drug used in hypertension

Atropine
An anticholinergic drug that has several uses – it can be used to reduce gastro-intestinal spasm, biliary and renal colic and in the treatment of bradycardia

Bendroflumethiazide
A thiazide diuretic used to treat congestive heart failure and hypertension

Benzylpenicillin
A penicillin antibiotic given by injection for the treatment of some infections

Bisoprolol fumarate
A beta-adrenoceptor blocking drug used in hypertension

Chlorpromazine
A neuroleptic drug used to reduce acute anxiety, as a pre-medication and in the management of terminal pain

Clopidogrel
An antiplatelet drug used to reduce the risk of clot (thrombus) formation in patients at risk

Dextrose 5%
An intravenous fluid containing dextrose

Dextrose 4% Saline 0.18%
An intravenous fluid used when dehydration is present but there is also a need for a source of energy

Diazepam
A benzodiazepine drug with anticonvulsant and anxiety-reducing effects

Diclofenac
A non-steroidal anti-inflammatory drug used to control pain and inflammation

Digoxin
A cardiac glycoside used to treat congestive heart failure and atrial fibrillation

Dihydrocodeine
A derivative of codeine used in the management of moderate to severe pain

Dopamine
A natural precursor of noradrenaline in the body, used to increase the force and rate of cardiac contraction and improve renal function in cardiogenic shock

Enoxaparin
A low molecular weight heparin used to treat or prevent thromboembolism

Epinephrine
A drug that mimics the effect of the sympathetic nervous system, used in anaphylactic shock

Ferrous fumarate
An iron solution used in iron deficiency anaemia

Furosemide

A powerful loop diuretic used to treat oedema

Gentamicin

An aminoglycoside antibiotic used in the treatment of severe infections

Gliclazide

A hypoglycaemic drug used in the management of Type 2 diabetes

Heparin

An anticoagulant drug used to treat thromboembolism

Hydrocortisone cream

A steroid-based cream used in itching skin conditions like eczema

Insulin

A replacement hormone used in the management of Type 1 and sometimes Type 2 diabetes

Irbesartan

An angiotensin receptor blocking drug used to treat high blood pressure

Lansoprazole

A drug used to reduce the amount of acid produced by the stomach

Levothyroxine sodium

A drug used to treat thyroid hormone deficiency in hypothyroidism

6-mercaptopurine

An antimetabolite drug used as chemotherapy in some malignant diseases

Metformin

A biguanide drug that is used in the management of Type 2 diabetes

Methotrexate

A cytotoxic drug with immunosuppressant activity

Metoprolol

A beta-adrenoceptor blocking drug used in hypertension

Midazolam

A drug used to produce sedation and amnesia

Morphine

A powerful narcotic drug used to control pain

Omeprazole

A drug used to reduce the amount of acid produced by the stomach

Oramorph
A morphine-based oral solution

Paracetamol
A commonly used mild analgesic drug

Penicillin V
An oral penicillin antibiotic used for the treatment of some infections

Perindopril
A long-acting angiotensin-converting enzyme (ACE) inhibitor used to treat high blood pressure

Potassium chloride
An intravenous drug used to correct electrolyte imbalance

Prednisolone
A steroid drug used to suppress inflammatory reactions in rheumatoid arthritis and asthma

Propranolol
A beta-adrenoceptor blocking drug used in hypertension

Ranitidine
A peptic ulcer healing drug

Ringer's solution
An intravenous fluid containing electrolytes

Sodium chloride 0.9%
An intravenous fluid used in fluid replacement

Sodium valproate
An anticonvulsant drug used in the management of epilepsy

Teicoplanin
An intravenous antibiotic used in the treatment of some severe infections

Warfarin
An oral anticoagulant drug used in the treatment and prevention of venous thrombosis and pulmonary embolism

Zopiclone
A drug used in the treatment of short-term insomnia

APPENDIX 5
MULTIPLICATION GRID

0	1	2	3	4	5	6	7	8	9	10	11	12
1	1	2	3	4	5	6	7	8	9	10	11	12
2	2	4	6	8	10	12	14	16	18	20	22	24
3	3	6	9	12	15	18	21	24	27	30	33	36
4	4	8	12	16	20	24	28	32	36	40	44	48
5	5	10	15	20	25	30	35	40	45	50	55	60
6	6	12	18	24	30	36	42	48	54	60	66	72
7	7	14	21	28	35	42	49	56	63	70	77	84
8	8	16	24	32	40	48	56	64	72	80	88	96
9	9	18	27	36	45	54	63	72	81	90	99	108
10	10	20	30	40	50	60	70	80	90	100	110	120
11	11	22	33	44	55	66	77	88	99	110	121	132
12	12	24	36	48	60	72	84	96	108	120	132	144

APPENDIX 6
CONVERSION TABLES

Weight conversions

METRIC (kg)	IMPERIAL (stones 'st' and pounds 'lb')	METRIC (kg)	IMPERIAL (stones 'st' and pounds 'lb')
50	7 st 12.2 lb	76	11 st 13.6 lb
52	8 st 2.6 lb	78	12 st 4 lb
54	8 st 7 lb	80	12 st 8.4 lb
56	8 st 11.5 lb	82	12 st 12.8 lb
58	9 st 1.9 lb	84	13 st 3.2 lb
60	9 st 6.3 lb	86	13 st 7.6 lb
62	9 st 10.7 lb	88	13 st 12 lb
64	10 st 1.1 lb	90	14 st 2.4 lb
66	10 st 5.5 lb	92	14 st 6.8 lb
68	10 st 9.9 lb	94	14 st 11.2 lb
70	11 st 0.3 lb	96	15 st 1.6 lb
72	11 st 4.7 lb	98	15 st 6.1 lb
74	11 st 9.1 lb	100	15 st 10.5 lb

Conversion formulae

To convert:

- kilograms to stones: multiply by 0.1575

- kilograms to pounds: multiply by 2.2046

- stones to kilograms: multiply by 6.3503

- pounds to kilograms: multiply by 0.4536

Height conversions

HEIGHT (FEET & INCHES)	HEIGHT (INCHES)	HEIGHT (METRES)	HEIGHT (CENTIMETRES)
4'	48	1.22	122
4'1"	49	1.24	124
4'2"	50	1.27	127
4'3"	51	1.29	129
4'4"	52	1.32	132
4'5"	53	1.35	135
4'6"	54	1.37	137
4'7"	55	1.4	140
4'8"	56	1.42	142
4'9"	57	1.45	145
4'10"	58	1.47	147
4'11"	59	1.5	150
5'	60	1.52	152
5'1"	61	1.55	155
5'2"	62	1.57	157
5'3"	63	1.6	160
5'4"	64	1.62	162
5'5"	65	1.65	165
5'6"	66	1.68	168
5'7"	67	1.7	170
5'8"	68	1.73	173
5'9"	69	1.75	175
5'10"	70	1.78	178
5'11"	71	1.8	180
6'	72	1.83	183

HEIGHT (FEET & INCHES)	HEIGHT (INCHES)	HEIGHT (METRES)	HEIGHT (CENTIMETRES)
6'1"	73	1.85	185
6'2"	74	1.88	188
6'3"	75	1.9	190
6'4"	76	1.93	193

(converted to the nearest centimetre)

Conversion formula

To convert:

- inches to centimetres: multiply by 2.54

ANSWERS TO SELF-ASSESSMENT TESTS

Test 1.1

1 59

2 One thousand and five

3 28 580

4 32

5 No units

6 45

7 7

8 161

9 Nine hundred and sixty thousand and twelve

10 48

11 29

12 Fifty thousands

13 108

14 1115

15 64%

16 252

17 No hundreds

18 14.375

19 650

20 8/10 or 4/5

21 3.8318

22 823 g

23 24

24 75

25 51.121064

26 1.189532

27 1200

28 ¾

29 0.55

30 6

Test 2.1: digit value

1   In the number 1.65, the digit '5' means five hundredths

2   In the number 6.079, the digit '0' means no tenths

3   In the number 8.125, the digit '5' means five thousandths

4   In the number 4012000, the digit '4' means four millions

5   In the number 12.75, the digit '2' means two ones

6   In the number 2.09, the digit '9' means nine hundredths

7   In the number 725.3, the digit '3' means three tenths

8   In the number 7.005, the digit '5' means five thousandths

9   In the number 0.13, the digit '3' means three hundredths

10 In the number 9.125, the digit '5' means five thousandths

Test 2.2: addition

1   23 + 77 = 100

2   156 + 239 = 395

3   17 + 3294 = 3311

4   21006 + 2005 = 23011

5   179 + 642 = 821

6   130 + 150 + 190 + 250 + 80 + 225 = 1025

7   125 + 145 + 155 + 68 + 95 + 300 = 888

8   500 + 200 + 150 + 45 + 60 + 120 + 397 = 1472

9   220 + 140 + 50 + 65 + 72 + 168 = 715

10 85 + 33 + 120 + 235 + 128 + 50 = 651

11 Total amount of fluid received = 675 ml

12 Total amount of fluid lost = 845 ml (chest drain 235 ml & vomit 610 ml)

Test 2.3: subtraction

1   155 – 42 = 113
2   1276 – 165 = 1111
3   916 – 817 = 99
4   96 – 58 = 38
5   117 – 99 = 18
6   2139 – 126 = 2013
7   6483 – 5261 = 1222
8   2912 – 1915 = 997
9   792 – 689 = 103
10   542 – 454 = 88
11   The overall fluid balance = 795 ml
12   There will be 40 ml left in the bottle

Test 2.4: multiplication

1   15 × 4 = 60
2   23 × 6 = 138
3   35 × 9 = 315
4   26 × 22 = 572
5   72 × 18 = 1296
6   124 × 12 = 1488
7   161 × 13 = 2093
8   148 × 17 = 2516
9   257 × 14 = 3598
10   321 × 67 = 21 507
11   Number of inhalations taken over 28 days = 112 so an inhaler containing 200 doses will be sufficient
12   50 ml need to be in the bottle to last until the patient returns

Test 2.5: multiplying decimals

1   Student Nurse Vipond will receive 6.375 hours of supervision from the lecturer
2   Student Nurse Jones is correct, she will manage to write 13.75 pages
3   1.875 L (0.75 × 2.5)
4   0.21 L (0.06 × 3.5)

5   3.125 kg (1.25 × 2.5)

6   1.125 L (0.25 × 4.5)

7   £262.80 (14.40 × 18.25)

Test 2.6: division

1   49 ÷ 7 = 7

2   84 ÷ 8 = 10.5

3   117 ÷ 9 = 13

4   72 ÷ 6 = 12

5   51 ÷ 4 = 12.75

6   87.5 ÷ 7 = 12.5

7   172 ÷ 8 = 21.5

8   67.5 ÷ 4 = 16.875

9   45 ÷ 6 = 7.5

10   130.5 ÷ 9 = 14.5

11   840 ÷ 8 = 105 ml/hr

12   96 ÷ 16 = 6 hours

Test 2.7: long division

1   846 ÷ 16 = 52.875

2   630 ÷ 15 = 42

3   1440 ÷ 12 = 120

4   702 ÷ 36 = 19.5

5   465.6 ÷ 24 = 19.4

6   188.1 ÷ 16 = 11.75625

7   1062.2 ÷ 47 = 22.6

8   719.2 ÷ 62 = 11.6

9   1093.75 ÷ 17.5 = 62.5

10   1163.75 ÷ 19 = 61.25

11   192 ÷ 16 = 12 days

12   182 ÷ 13 = 14 days

Test 2.8: percentages

1 $\dfrac{36}{45} \times 100 = 80\%$ of the patients are female

2 $\dfrac{10030}{50150} \times 100 = 20\%$ of the patients are children

3 $\dfrac{14}{56} \times 100 = 25\%$ of the residents are male

4 $\dfrac{7}{72} \times 100 = 9.72\%$ are arterial ulcers

5 $\dfrac{65}{245} \times 100 = 26.53\%$ did not require hospital transport

6 $\dfrac{169}{496} \times 100 = 34.07\%$ did not need aftercare

7 $\dfrac{39}{326} \times 100 = 11.96\%$ of the patients did not attend for screening

8 $\dfrac{56}{200} \times 100 = 28\%$ of the patients had sutures

9 There is a 44.44% increase in the pulse rate

10 There is a 15% increase in the peak expiratory flow rate

Test 2.9: summary test

1 In the number 84 938, the digit '4' means four thousands

2 In the number 2971.03, the digit '3' means three hundredths

3 In the number 1 269 351, the digit '6' means sixty thousands

4 150 + 75 + 225 + 345 + 63 + 99 = 957

5 180 + 60 + 193 + 2025 + 55 + 120 + 94 = 2727

6 220 + 30 + 960 + 710 + 1203 + 328 + 415 = 3866

7 67 + 53 + 89 + 239 + 421 + 917 + 1501 + 27 = 3314

8 862 − 771 = 91

9 1915 − 907 = 1008

10 491 − 269 = 222

11 26 × 19 = 494

12 127 × 16 = 2032

13 132 × 112 = 14784

14 179 × 235 = 42 065

15 6.7 × 4.2 = 28.14

16 69.72 × 1.13 = 78.7836

17 54.176 × 2.05 = 111.0608

18 27.147 × 5.628 = 152.783316

19 114 ÷ 8 = 14.25

20 295.2 ÷ 12 = 24.6

21 1201.2 ÷ 21 = 57.2

22 168 ÷ 19.2 = 8.75

23 Factors of 24 are: 1, 2, 3, 4, 6, 8, 12 & 24

24 Factors of 39 are: 1, 3, 13 & 39

25 Factors of 66 are: 1, 2, 3, 6, 11, 22, 33 & 66

26 Factors of 82 are: 1, 2, 41 & 82

27 Factors of 90 are: 1, 2, 3, 5, 6, 9, 10, 15, 18, 30, 45 & 90

28 31.25% of patients needed the assessment

29 5% did not attend

30 7.5% needed additional advice

Test 3.1: converting kilograms and grams

1 There are 1300 g in 1.3 kg

2 There are 1250 g in 1.25 kg

3 There are 800 g in 0.8 kg

4 There are 125 g in 0.125 kg

5 There are 1204 g in 1.204 kg

6 There are 500 g in 0.5 kg

7 There are 2030 g in 2.03 kg

8 There are 32 g in 0.032 kg

9 There are 1005 g in 1.005 kg

10 There are 2 g in 0.002 kg

11 There are 2.5 kg in 2500 g

12 There are 4.025 kg in 4025 g

13 There are 0.75 kg in 750 g

14 The scale indicates 100 g

15 The scale indicates 800 g

Test 3.2: converting grams and milligrams

1 There are 1040 mg in 1.04 g

2 There are 1005 mg in 1.005 g

3 There is 1 mg in 0.001 g

4 There are 2202 mg in 2.202 g

5 There are 1016 mg in 1.016 g

6 There are 330 mg in 0.33 g

7 There are 750 mg in 0.75 g

8 There are 60 mg in 0.06 g

9 There are 1018 mg in 1.018 g

10 There are 106 mg in 0.106 g

11 There are 1.5 g in 1500 mg

12 There are 2.2 g in 2200 mg

13 There are 0.9 g in 900 mg

14 0.85 g

15 0.625 g

Test 3.3: converting milligrams and micrograms

1 There are 1250 micrograms in 1.25 mg

2 There are 1062 micrograms in 1.062 mg

3 There are 75 micrograms in 0.075 mg

4 There are 220 micrograms in 0.220 mg

5 There are 1028 micrograms in 1.028 mg

6 There are 9 micrograms in 0.009 mg

7 There are 700 micrograms in 0.7 mg

8 There are 125 micrograms in 0.125 mg

9 There are 1500 micrograms in 1.5 mg

10 There are 750 micrograms in 0.75 mg

11 There are 1.2 milligrams in 1200 micrograms

12 There are 0.8 milligrams in 800 micrograms

13 There are 0.25 milligrams in 250 micrograms

14 Each inhalation is 0.1 milligrams

15 There are 600 micrograms in 0.6 milligrams

Test 3.4: summary test

1   There are 1300 mg in 1.3 g

2   There are 800 mg in 0.8 g

3   There are 1125 mg in 1.125 g

4   There are 600 mg in 0.6 g

5   There are 505 mg in 0.505 g

6   There are 750 micrograms in 0.75 mg

7   There are 1001 micrograms in 1.001 mg

8   There are 70 micrograms in 0.07 mg

9   There are 902 micrograms in 0.902 mg

10   There are 1500 millilitres in 1.5 L

11   There are 2250 millilitres in 2.25 L

12   There are 100 millilitres in 0.1 L

13   There are 75 millilitres in 0.075 L

14   There are 5 millilitres in 0.005 L

15   The syringe contains 0.7 ml

16   The medicine pot contains 12 ml

17   The completed table should look like this:

GRAMS (g)	MILLIGRAMS (mg)	MICROGRAMS
0.006	6	6000
0.00012	0.120	120
0.01	10	10 000
0.0095	9.5	9500
1	1000	1 000 000
0.00025	0.25	250
0.001	1	1000
0.00275	2.75	2750
0.008	8	8000
0.0005	0.5	500

18   22.5 mg + 4600 micrograms = 27.1 mg

19   1.6 mg + 500 micrograms = 2.1 mg

20   4.005 mg + 6 micrograms = 4.011 mg

21 123 mg – 900 micrograms = 122.1 mg

22 6 mg – 25 micrograms = 5.975 mg

23 The correct order is:
3 micrograms, 0.005 mg (5 micrograms), 25 micrograms, 0.034 mg
(34 micrograms), 65 micrograms, 0.25 mg (250 micrograms), 400 micrograms,
1100 micrograms (1.1 mg), 1.5 mg, 1.6 mg, 1607 micrograms, 5 mg,
0.065 g (65 mg), 0.125 g (125 mg), 200 mg, 0.22 g (220 mg), 0.5 g (500 mg),
750 mg, 1.5 g, 2 g, 2100 mg (2.1 g)

24 The patient takes 1.05 g per day

25 **a** There are 30 mg in 7.5 ml

 b There are 50 mg in 12.5 ml

26 1000 micrograms

27 0.4 mg

28 1500 mg

29 0.3 g

30 5000 micrograms

Test 4.1: calculating tablets

1 2

2 3

3 0.5

4 2

5 Gliclazide 40 mg in the morning of 08/02

6 Metoprolol 50 mg at bedtime on 15/02

7 The correct dose is between 100 and 250 micrograms

8 The prescription does need to be checked with the prescriber as the drug is
night sedation and usually given at bedtime

Test 4.2: calculating liquid medicines

1 10 ml

2 10 ml

3 15 ml

4 20 ml

5 Diazepam oral solution, 4 mg (10 ml) at midday on 22/09

6 15 ml

7   10 ml is the appropriate dose once or twice daily before food

8   The prescription needs checking with the prescriber as a very low dose has been prescribed. Initially 80 mg twice daily can be given increasing to 320 mg per day

Test 4.3: calculating injections

1   2 ml

2   2.5 ml

3   1.5 ml

4   2 ml

5   Furosemide 25 mg, 2.5 ml

6   Dihydrocodeine 40 mg, 0.8 ml

7   5 ampoules are needed for the 3 mg dose. The usual dose is between 300 micrograms and 1 mg (1000 micrograms)

8   Yes, the prescription needs checking with the prescriber as the usual dose is between 100 and 500 mg, three or four times in 24 hours

Test 4.4: calculating intravenous flow rates

1   125 ml/hr

2   250 ml/hr

3   125 ml/hr

4   312.5 ml are still to be infused after 3 hours. 187.5 ml have been infused

5   150 ml are still to be infused after 7 hours. 350 ml have been infused

6   375 ml are still to be infused after 5 hours. 625 ml have been infused

7   200 ml are still to be infused after 3 hours. 300 ml have been infused

8   750 ml have been infused after 6 hours. 250 ml are still to be infused

9   125 ml have been infused after 1 hour. 375 ml are still to be infused

10   625 ml have been infused after 2.5 hours. 375 ml are still to be infused

Test 4.5: calculating intravenous infusion drop rates

1   55.5r drops per minute is the answer but 55 drops per minute is used to avoid air entering the intravenous giving set

2   55.5r drops per minute is the answer but 55 drops per minute is used to avoid air entering the intravenous giving set

3   33.3r drops per minute is the answer but 33 drops per minute is used to avoid air entering the intravenous giving set

4 83.3r drops per minute is the answer but 83 drops per minute is used to avoid air entering the intravenous giving set

5 41.6r drops per minute is the answer but 41 drops per minute is used to avoid air entering the intravenous giving set

6 41.6r drops per minute is the answer but 41 drops per minute is used to avoid air entering the intravenous giving set

7 27.7r drops per minute is the answer but 27 drops per minute is used to avoid air entering the intravenous giving set

8 The method used to calculate the new drop rate is:

- Firstly identify the volume of fluid that has been infused

- Input the new (remaining) volume and new timescale into the equation:

$$\frac{\text{Volume prescribed (ml)}}{\text{Hours of infusion}} \times \frac{\text{Drops per ml of administration set}}{60 \text{ minutes}}$$

After 3 hours half of the fluid (250 ml) has been infused, as the original prescription was 500 ml over 6 hours, so these new values need to go into the equation:

- Remaining fluid = 250 ml

- New timescale = 2 hours

$$\frac{250}{2} \times \frac{20}{60} = 41 \text{ drops per minute (rounded down from 41.6)}$$

9 The method used to calculate the new drop rate is the same as for Question 8.

After 4.5 hours, half of the fluid (500 ml) has been infused, as the original prescription was 1000 ml over 9 hours, so these new values need to go into the equation:

- Remaining fluid = 500 ml

- New timescale = 3 hours

$$\frac{500}{3} \times \frac{20}{60} = 55 \text{ drops per minute (rounded down from 55.5)}$$

10 The method used to calculate the new drop rate is the same as for Question 8.

After 1 hour, only 50 ml of the fluid has been infused. The original volume was 500 ml over 10 hours, which gives an hourly rate of 50 ml (500 ÷ 10 = 50 ml per hour) so these new values need to go into the equation:

- Remaining fluid = 450 ml

- New timescale = 5 hours

$$\frac{450}{5} \times \frac{20}{60} = 30 \text{ drops per minute}$$

11 41.6r drops per minute is the answer but 41 drops per minute is used to avoid air entering the intravenous giving set

12 31.25 drops per minute is the answer but 31 drops per minute is used to avoid air entering the intravenous giving set

Test 4.6: calculating dose per kilogram of body weight

1 a 360 mg   b 120 mg
2 a 75 mg   b 25 mg
3 a 12900 micrograms   b 12.9 mg
4 a 5600 micrograms   b 5.6 mg
5 a 340 micrograms   b 12.24 ml

Test 4.7: summary test

1   2 tablets
2   1.5 tablets
3   2 tablets
4   2 tablets
5   2 tablets
6   7.5 ml
7   10 ml
8   1.5 ml
9   7.5 ml
10 2.5 ml
11 4 ml
12 2 ml
13 1.2 ml
14 0.8 ml
15 0.7 ml
16 133 ml/hr
17 55 dpm
18 250 ml/hr
19 83 dpm
20 125 ml/hr
21 41 dpm

22 125 ml/hr

23 27 dpm

24 111 ml/hr

25 83 dpm

26 380 micrograms

27 6000 micrograms or 6 mg

28 10 500 units

29 1700 micrograms or 1.7 mg

30 420 mg

31 3700 micrograms or 3.7 mg

32 28 800 micrograms or 28.8 mg

33 10 200 micrograms or 10.2 mg

34 a   The dose per minute = 375 micrograms.

    b   The dose over one hour = 22 500 micrograms or 22.5 mg

Test 5.1: fluid balance chart (1)

1 The total oral intake = 1400 ml

2 The total intravenous intake = 1000 ml

3 The total fluid intake = 2400 ml

4 The total urine output = 2700 ml

5 The total fluid output = 2700 ml

6 The fluid balance for this 24-hour period = –300 ml

Test 5.2: fluid balance chart (2)

1 The total oral intake = 2000 ml

2 The total intravenous intake = 500 ml

3 The total fluid intake = 2500 ml

4 The total urine output = 2700 ml

5 The total fluid output = 2900 ml

6 The fluid balance for this 24-hour period = –400 ml

Test 5.3: calculating BMI

1 BMI = 28.2

2 BMI = 20.7

3 BMI = 19.9

4 BMI = 24.8

5 BMI = 26.6

6 BMI = 31.2 Weight status: obese

7 BMI = 26.9 Weight status: overweight

8 BMI = 24.7 Weight status: normal

9 BMI = 24.6 Weight status: normal

10 BMI = 28.7 Weight status: overweight

Test 5.4: 'MUST' score risk calculations

1 BMI: 29.7 Weight loss: 4.9% Risk: 2/High

2 BMI: 20.5 Weight loss: 7.5% Risk: 3/High

3 BMI: 20.3 Weight loss: 9.7% Risk: 1/Medium

4 BMI: 20.7 Weight loss: 7.6% Risk: 1/Medium

5 BMI: 19.9 Weight loss: 8.1% Risk: 2/High

6 BMI: 22.7 Weight loss: 0% Risk: 0/Low

7 BMI: 30.9 Weight loss: 0% Risk: 0/Low

8 BMI: 21 Weight loss: 0% Risk: 2/High

9 BMI: 29.6 Weight loss: 0% Risk: 0/Low

10 BMI: 23.7 Weight loss: 0% Risk: 2/High

Test 5.5: ideal body weight

1 The ideal body weight for a male, 1.67 m tall is 63 kg

2 The ideal body weight for a female, 1.545 m tall is 47.8 kg

3 The ideal body weight for a male, 1.7 m tall is 66 kg

4 The ideal body weight for a female, 1.68 m tall is 60.2 kg

5 The ideal body weight for a male, 1.87 m tall is 83 kg

6 The ideal body weight for a female, 1.6 m tall is 52.9 kg

7 The ideal body weight for a male, 1.77 m tall is 73 kg

8 The ideal body weight for a female, 1.62 m tall is 54.7 kg

9 The ideal body weight for a male, 1.72 m tall is 68 kg

10 The ideal body weight for a female, 1.57 m tall is 50.1 kg

Test 6.1: working in SI units (1)

1   0.025 mg = 25 micrograms

2   0.601 mg = 601 micrograms

3   0.909 mg = 909 micrograms

4   1.005 mg = 1005 micrograms

5   1.2 mg = 1200 micrograms

6   0.25 L = 250 ml

7   0.905 L = 905 ml

8   0.02 L = 20 ml

9   0.3 L = 300 ml

10   0.075 L = 75 ml

11   1 microgram = 0.001 mg

12   1 kg = 1 000 000 mg

13   500 micrograms = 0.5 mg

14   1.2 g = 1200 mg

15   75 micrograms = 0.075 mg

16   750 micrograms – 0.25 mg = 500 micrograms

17   5 micrograms + 0.05 mg = 55 micrograms

18   1.029 mg – 290 micrograms = 739 micrograms

19   1.1 g + 10 mg = 1.11 g

20   0.75 g – 500 mg = 250 mg

Test 6.2: working in SI units (2)

1   0.0056 mg = 5.6 micrograms

2   1.01 mg = 1010 micrograms

3   2 mg = 2000 micrograms

4   1 g = 1 000 000 micrograms

5   3.005 mg = 3005 micrograms

6   0.05 L = 50 ml

7   1.002 L = 1002 ml

8   1.6 L = 1600 ml

9   0.009 L = 9 ml

10   0.106 L = 106 ml

11 1.5 g = 1500 mg

12 25 micrograms = 0.025 mg

13 5 micrograms = 0.005 mg

14 2.01 g = 2010 mg

15 0.032 g = 32 mg

16 16 micrograms + 0.999 mg = 1.015 mg

17 1002 micrograms – 0.02 mg = 982 micrograms

18 1 g – 5 mg = 995 mg

19 995 mg + 0.005 g = 1 g

20 890 mg + 0.111 g = 1.001 g

Test 6.3: working in SI units (3)

1 0.35 mg = 350 micrograms

2 3 mg = 3000 micrograms

3 2.002 mg = 2002 micrograms

4 0.006 mg = 6 micrograms

5 0.75 g = 750 000 micrograms

6 0.75 L = 750 ml

7 1.03 L = 1030 ml

8 0.005 L = 5 ml

9 0.04 L = 40 ml

10 2.02 L = 2020 ml

11 2.2 g = 2200 mg

12 6 micrograms = 0.006 mg

13 0.02 g = 20 mg

14 65 micrograms = 0.065 mg

15 0.8 kg = 800 000 mg

16 0.9 g – 8 mg = 892 mg

17 0.08 mg + 15 micrograms = 95 micrograms

18 1.2 mg – 400 micrograms = 800 micrograms

19 0.75 mg + 300 micrograms = 1.05 mg

20 75 mg + 0.005 g = 80 mg

Test 6.4: calculating drug doses (1)

1. 3
2. 1.5
3. 5
4. 0.5
5. 3
6. 2.5
7. 2
8. 2
9. 6
10. 3
11. 5 ml
12. 1152 mg
13. 180 mg
14. 528 mg
15. 225 mg
16. 2 ml
17. 1.5 ml
18. 4.4 ml
19. 3 ml
20. 3 ml

Test 6.5: calculating drug doses (2)

1. 5
2. 0.5
3. 2.5
4. 3
5. 0.5
6. 2
7. 4
8. 3
9. 4
10. 1.5

11 15 ml

12 204 mg

13 270 mg

14 300 mg

15 864 mg

16 3 ml

17 0.5 ml

18 2.5 ml

19 1.6 ml

20 2.5 ml

Test 6.6: Calculating drug doses (3)

1 2

2 4

3 3

4 3

5 2

6 4

7 3

8 2

9 4

10 3

11 5 ml

12 20 ml

13 340 mg

14 200 mg

15 144 mg

16 0.5 ml

17 1.5 ml

18 0.5 ml

19 2.5 ml

20 1.25 ml

Test 6.7

1 0.009 mg = 9 micrograms

2 0.057 mg = 57 micrograms

3 0.248 L = 248 ml

4 0.002 L = 2 ml

5 6 micrograms = 0.006 mg

6 2.3 g = 2300 mg

7 3

8 2

9 30 ml

10 2.2 ml

11 4.2 ml

12 1.7 ml

13 0.55 ml

14 2.4 ml

15 1.1 ml

16 6 ml

17 10 ml

18 21 ml

19 False, it is due on the 22/10

20 True

21 True

22 False, it is for Chloe Edwards

23 False, four 5 mg tablets are due

24 No Dr's signature for co-codamol 30/500
No start date for amoxicillin
Patient allergic to penicillin, yet amoxicillin prescribed
Combination of co-codamol 30/500 and paracetamol would result
 in a serious overdose
Amoxicillin dose should be 8 hourly
Paracetamol, no start date
Paracetamol, no route specified

Test 6.8

1 0.306 mg = 306 micrograms

2 0.001 mg = 1 microgram

3 0.407 L = 407 ml

4 2.02 L = 2020 ml

5 600 micrograms = 0.6 mg

6 72 micrograms = 0.072 mg

7 2.5

8 3

9 330 mg

10 0.5 ml

11 3.2 ml

12 0.35 ml

13 1.8 ml

14 0.95 ml

15 1.3 ml

16 14 ml

17 8 ml

18 17 ml

19 False, the total amount of paracetamol taken over seven days will be 28 g

20 False, the next dose of nitrofurantoin is 50 mg at midday on 29/07

21 True

22 False, the next dose of paracetamol due at midday on 29/07 is two 500 mg tablets

23 True

24 There is no information about allergies that the patient may have
There is no name on the prescription
Phenytoin is suspension, yet the route indicates intravenously
Digoxin is written in milligrams, not micrograms
There is no start date for the digoxin
The maximum dosage for paracetamol is 4 g daily, yet the prescription states
    6 g per day
The paracetamol prescription is not signed

Test 6.9

1 2.022 mg = 2022 micrograms

2 0.101 mg = 101 micrograms

3 0.082 L = 82 ml

4 2.01 L = 2010 ml

5 0.053 g = 53 mg

6 9 micrograms = 0.009 mg

7 3

8 2

9 384 mg

10 2.5 ml

11 0.65 ml

12 3.6 ml

13 1.6 ml

14 4.8 ml

15 0.5 ml

16 18 ml

17 9 ml

18 13 ml

19 False, the patient takes 1.5 g of metformin over each 24-hour period

20 False, he is allergic to trimethoprim

21 True

22 True

23 False, atenolol 50 mg is next due on 23/09

24 The digoxin is prescribed twice daily but is normally only taken once daily

The digoxin has no prescriber's signature

There is no start date for the simvastatin

There is no prescriber's signature for the simvastatin

400 mg simvastatin is prescribed; 40 mg is a normal dose

There is no route specified for the furosemide

Furosemide is not routinely given at bedtime as it will cause sleep disturbance

Test 6.10

1 0.275 mg = 275 micrograms

2 0.016 mg = 16 micrograms

3 0.072 L = 72 ml

4 0.902 L = 902 ml

5 1.25 g = 1250 mg

6 35 micrograms = 0.035 mg

7 3

8 2

9 225 mg

10 1.5 ml

11 2.8 ml

12 1.4 ml

13 0.65 ml

14 4.4 ml

15 1.6 ml

16 22 ml

17 16 ml

18 7 ml

19 False, the next dose of irbesartan is for one 300 mg tablet on the morning of 23/10

20 False, clopidogrel 75 mg, to be given in the morning, is prescribed daily

21 True

22 False, the patient's next dose of lansoprazole is for 30 mg on the morning of 23/10

23 8.75 mg

24 2.1 g

25 No patient date of birth on the prescription

No route of administration given for perindopril

No prescription start date for amlodipine

Prescription for amlodipine not signed by a doctor

No route identified for omeprazole

Very high dose of omeprazole; usually starts at 10–20 mg, usually given once daily

REFERENCES

BAPEN (2012) *Malnutrition Matters: meeting quality standards in nutritional care.* Available at tinyurl.com/p776wjs (accessed 30 October 2019)

Charani, E. *et al.* (2015) Lack of weight recording in patients being administered narrow therapeutic index antibiotics: a prospective cross-sectional study. *BMJ Open,* **5:e**006092. Available at tinyurl.com/y29jaaqp (accessed 30 October 2019)

Francis, R. (chair) (2013) *Report of the Mid Staffordshire NHS Foundation Trust Public Inquiry.* The Stationery Office. Available at tinyurl.com/y4jz3c3u (accessed 30 October 2019)

Griffiths, P. and Jull, A. (2010) How good is the evidence for using risk assessment to prevent pressure ulcers?, nursingtimes.net April 12, 2010. Available at tinyurl.com/jybcxm2 (accessed 30 October 2019)

ISMP Canada (2016) *Weight-Based Medication Dose Errors.* Available at tinyurl.com/y276rp7r (accessed 30 October 2019)

Keers, R.N., Williams, S.D., Cooke, J. and Ashcroft, D.M. (2013) Prevalence and nature of medication administration errors in health care settings: a systematic review of direct observational evidence. *Annals of Pharmacotherapy,* **47**: 237–56.

Nightingale, F. (1859) (reprinted 1970) *Notes on Nursing: what it is and what it is not.* Blackie.

NPSA (2010) National Patient Safety Agency Rapid Response Report RRR014. Available at tinyurl.com/y2jnskds (accessed 30 October 2019)

Nursing & Midwifery Council (2018) *Future Nurse: standards of proficiency for registered nurses.* Available at tinyurl.com/yywjl8nt (accessed 30 October 2019)